D1433938

Percutaneous Tracheostomy
A Practical Handbook

Percutaneous Tracheostomy
A Practical Handbook

Henry G.W. Paw BPharm MRPharmS MBBS FRCA
Consultant in Anaesthesia and Intensive Care

York Hospital, York, UK

Andrew R. Bodenham MBBS FRCA
Consultant in Anaesthesia and Intensive Care

Leeds General Infirmary, Leeds, UK

Project Manager
Gavin Smith, GPS Publishing Solutions

Typeset by Charon Tec Pvt. Ltd, Chennai, India

Printed and bound in the UK by Cambridge University Press

Contents

Preface

Percutaneous tracheostomy is now a standard technique in many intensive care units worldwide. It has completed the range of airway techniques available to anaesthetists and intensivists and transformed practice for both intensive care staff and more importantly the patients.

Some 15 years ago (late 1980s) whilst still a trainee, one of the authors (Andrew R. Bodenham) set out to learn open surgical tracheostomy techniques as he was fed up with delays and problems in getting tracheostomies done in a timely fashion in patients requiring intensive care. At the same time percutaneous tracheostomy kits were just reaching the market place. Armed with a video of the Ciaglia technique and somewhat sceptical support from local ear, nose and throat (ENT) surgeons, a case was set up in the ENT theatre, with the ENT registrar for support and three consultant ENT surgeons watching. The needle, cannula and guidewire were passed blindly into the trachea without incident but successive dilators produced increasing volumes of venous blood from the stoma. The percutaneous technique was converted to an open procedure and completed without further problems. The guidewire was seen to have transfixed a large midline anterior jugular vein. This was one of the first such procedures in the UK and certainly the first failure. Other successful procedures followed without incident despite widespread doubts from colleagues. The rest is history! We suspect many others have had similar experiences.

There are now many different kits and techniques and it is likely that further developments will expand the role of such devices into anaesthesia, elective surgery and emergency airway practice. A generation of trainees are now coming through with such skills. There are still concerns about the overall safety of such techniques in particular as the numbers of procedures increase on a year-by-year basis.

In this book we have tried to present a balanced overview of techniques without getting overwhelmed with detail.

Henry G.W. Paw
Andrew R. Bodenham
2004

Acknowledgements

To my wife, Leonie, and my children, Matthew and Georgina, for their encouragement, understanding and love.

To Mike Pringle and Alan Pettigrew from the Medical Illustration Department at York Hospital.

Henry G.W. Paw

Thanks to family, friends and colleagues for their continuing interest and support over the years.

Andrew R. Bodenham

Abbreviations

BP	Blood pressure
COPD	Chronic obstructive pulmonary disease
CPAP	Continuous positive airway pressure
CT	Computed tomography
ECG	Electrocardiogram
ENT	Ear, nose and throat
ET tube	Endotracheal tube
$ETCO_2$	End tidal CO_2
FG	French gauge
FiO_2	Fractional inspired oxygen
FRC	Functional residual capacity
GI	Gastrointestinal
h	Hour
HDU	High dependency unit
HME	Heat moisture exchange
ICP	Intracranial pressure
ICU	Intensive care unit
ID	Internal diameter
INR	International normalised ratio
IPPV	Intermittent positive pressure ventilation
kg	Kilogram
LMA	Laryngeal mask airway
min	Minute
MRI	Magnetic resonance imaging
MRSA	Methicillin-resistant *Staphylococcus aureus*
NG	Nasogastric
$PaCO_2$	Partial pressure of carbon dioxide in arterial blood
PaO_2	Partial pressure of oxygen in arterial blood
PEEP	Positive end expiratory pressure
PcT	Percutaneous tracheostomy
s	Second
SaO_2	Arterial oxygen saturation
USS	Ultrasound scan

History of Tracheostomy

Early references

The earliest known references to tracheostomy were made in the
Rigveda, a sacred Hindu book published around 2000 BC.[1] The
surgical procedure of tracheostomy is thought to be portrayed on
Egyptian wooden tablets dating back to around 3000 BC.[2] Two tablets
were discovered dating from the beginning of the first
dynasty, one in Abydos concerning King Aha (Figure 1.1) and the
other in Saqqara, concerning King Djer (Figure 1.2). Each tablet
depicts a seated person directing a pointed instrument to the throat of
another person who is leaning backwards. Some experts believed
that this denotes human sacrifice whereas others believe it to be a
tracheostomy or other surgical procedure. Ankh, the sign of life
(Figure 1.3) is seen in this tablet, in which a God presents life to a King.
The same sign is present in Aha's tablet, above the heads of both
operator and patient, signifying that life is given from one to the other.
The way the scalpel is handled suggests that it is more appropriately
directed to the trachea than the neck vessels. The arms placed behind

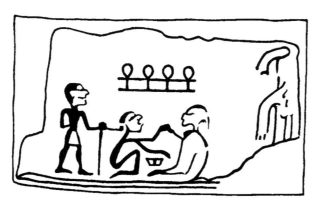

Fig. 1.1 **King Aha
tablet – tracheostomy,
first dynasty.**

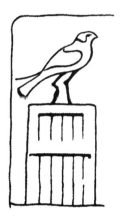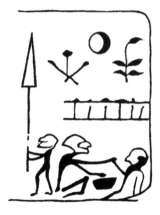

Fig. 1.2 King Djer tablet – tracheostomy, first dynasty.

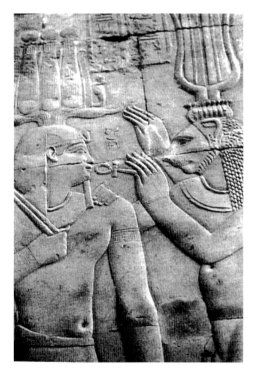

Fig. 1.3 Ankh, sign of life, presented by a God to a King.

the person operated upon can be explained in terms of the modern practice of placing a sandbag between the shoulder blades of patients undergoing tracheostomy. It is of note that most authorities believe that human sacrifice was not practised in ancient Egypt.

In the Roman era, tracheostomies were performed using a large incision and a warning was given that it was dangerous to divide the whole trachea.[3]

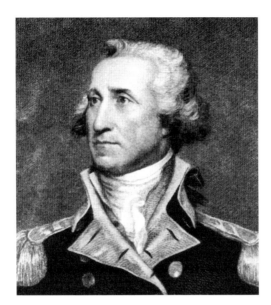

Fig. 1.4 George Washington, 1732–1799.

In the middle ages, there were sporadic reports of such procedures, but the history of surgical access to the airway was largely one of condemnation. The technique of slashing the throat to save life was known as 'semislaughter'.

During the Renaissance, most surgeons were reluctant to perform the procedure, even after the Italian Antonio Musa Brasavola's (1500–1570) report of a successful tracheostomy.[4]

One cold December afternoon in the year 1799, in Virginia, USA, three physicians were gathered around a dying man. The man was gasping for air, so the physicians gave him sage tea with vinegar to gargle, but this almost choked him. The patient's airway was severely compromised. It had been only a year since the medical literature of the time had described a surgical procedure in which the trachea could be accessed in cases of upper airway obstruction. Before 1800, elective or emergency tracheostomy was rarely performed. The patient's condition continued to deteriorate as he struggled for breath. One of the physicians was aware of the tracheostomy procedure described earlier in the literature but was reluctant to attempt it on such a famous person. After a short time, the patient became calm and died. Historians may recognise this story as that of George Washington (Figure 1.4). The most popular theory is that he

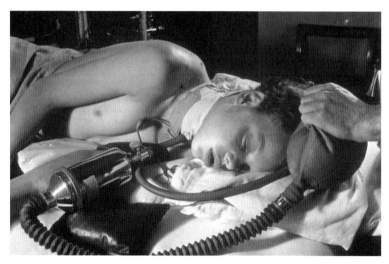

Fig. 1.5 **Boy with tetanus in Leeds unit, 1950s.**

died from an upper airway obstruction caused by bacterial epiglottitis.[5] Perhaps if a tracheostomy procedure had been successfully performed, it would have popularised the technique earlier.

In the early 1800s, it became more common for children to receive tracheostomies as a treatment for advanced diphtheria. Modern open surgical tracheostomy techniques were standardised in 1909 by Chevalier Jackson.[6]

In the early days of intensive care (Figure 1.5), including the Scandinavian poliomyelitis epidemics of the 1950s, tracheostomy become the accepted means of airway management for the provision of long-term ventilation.[7] Thereafter, there were few changes in surgical techniques until the introduction of percutaneous tracheostomy.

Development of percutaneous tracheostomy

There were devices available historically to facilitate rapid percutaneous tracheostomy but without the benefit of guidewires and flexible dilators/introducers. Such devices were inherently unsafe and never achieved widespread usage. The Italian surgeon Sanctorio Sanctorius (1561–1636), a professor at the University of Padua, was probably the first surgeon to describe percutaneous tracheostomy.

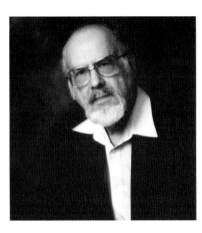

Fig. 1.6 Pasquale Ciaglia, 1912–2001.

Sanctorius described the procedure in his book[8] but does not seem to have performed it himself.[3]

The term percutaneous tracheostomy was first used by Shelden in 1955.[9] To minimise the risk of damaging vital structures, Shelden first introduced a slot-needle into the tracheal lumen. He loaded the cannula onto a cutting trocar, slid it along the slot and then introduced it into the tracheal lumen. In 1969, Toye and Weinstein used a Seldinger guidewire to allow the safe introduction of a cannula, providing a vital step towards popularisation of percutaneous techniques.[10]

Pasquale Ciaglia (Figure 1.6), a thoracic surgeon at St Elizabeth Hospital, New York, was concerned about tracheal stenosis from surgical tracheostomy. Encouraged by work done by Brantigan and Grow in 1976[11] on cricothyroidotomy, Ciaglia first developed subcricoid fingertip tracheostomy before moving on to full percutaneous tracheostomy, where the only incision needed is to the skin to admit the index finger for palpation of the cartilages. He reported the first percutaneous progressive dilatational technique in June 1985 on a series of 26 patients.[12] He used a modified percutaneous nephrostomy set to perform the tracheostomy.

Early results were excellent, comparing favourably with open surgical techniques. The technique gained popularity in 1990 with the availability of a commercial kit produced by Cook® Critical Care Products. The first use in the UK was in January 1990 by Leinhardt and Mughal, of the University Department of Surgery at Hope

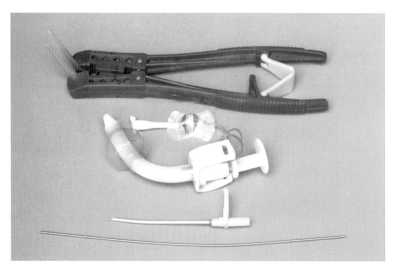

Fig. 1.7 Rapitrach (Surgitech, Sydney, Australia).

Hospital, Salford. Other units soon followed.[13] The use of percutaneous tracheostomy quickly spread throughout the UK, making it a European leader in the use of the technique. Since then, numerous authors have supported the findings of the pioneers of the technique. Others have reported additions to further improve the technique, such as bronchoscopy guidance and the use of ultrasound.

Schachner described an alternative technique, the Rapitrach kit (Figure 1.7) in 1989. This involved placing a guidewire into the tracheal lumen, followed by the passage of a short-jawed metal tracheotome. This was opened in the trachea, allowing a tracheostomy tube to be inserted between the open jaws of the instrument.[14] This device was originally designed for emergency use, providing rapid access to the trachea. However, the forceps, when opened, often lay in the pretracheal tissues, the sharp bevelled tip was associated with rupture of the tracheostomy tube cuff and there were reports of posterior tracheal wall damage. As a result of such complications, some resulting in death, it is no longer widely used. The Percutrac[15] was a minor modification of the Rapitrach, designed to be reusable (Figure 1.8). The longer jaws were designed to make pretracheal placement less likely.

In 1990, Griggs described an alternative technique using a pair of dilating forceps.[16] This is marketed by Portex in the UK.

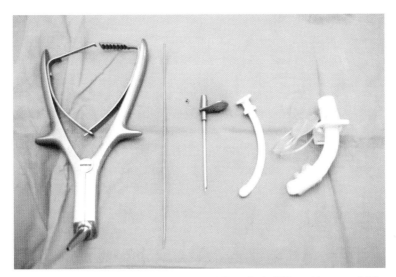

Fig. 1.8 Percutrac (John Weiss and Son Ltd, Milton Keynes, UK).

In 1997, Fantoni described the translaryngeal approach. This was a new approach where the tracheostomy tube was pulled from inside the trachea to the outside.[17]

In 1999 (before his death in June 2001, aged 89), Ciaglia further modified his original sequential dilatational technique into a one-step dilatational technique with the Blue Rhino kit. This is said to have a number of advantages over the original kit, including the use of a softer hydrophilic coated single-step dilator.[18] In 2001, Portex brought out a similar kit with a white single stage dilator.

The latest modification to percutaneous tracheostomy kits comes in the form of the PercuTwist developed by Rüsch in 2002.[19] The screw-tipped dilator is claimed to offer more controlled dilation of the trachea.

There have been parallel developments of other devices utilising similar principles (e.g. the Minitrach Seldinger and Melker emergency cricothyroidotomy kit). The so-called minitracheostomy technique was first described in 1984[20] and subsequently modified into a Seldinger technique.[21] Such techniques appear to be used less frequently since the advent of larger-bore percutaneous tracheostomy sets.

A recent survey showed that percutaneous tracheostomy is performed in 75% of intensive care units in England and Wales, making bedside percutaneous tracheostomy the technique of choice for patients requiring tracheostomy.[22] The most commonly used kit in the survey was the original Cook Ciaglia kit (46.6%), followed by the latest Cook Blue Rhino kit (31.3%), which appears to be increasing in popularity. The routine use of fibreoptic bronchoscopy guidance has increased from 30% in 1998[23] to 80.6% in 2002. However, capnography was only used in 1.2% of the ICUs.

References

1　Frost EAM. Tracing the tracheostomy. *Ann Otol Rhinol Laryngol* 1976; **85**: 618

2　Pahor AL. Ear, nose and throat in Ancient Egypt. *J Laryngol Otol* 1992; **106**: 773–9

3　van Heurn LWE, Brink PRG. The history of percutaneous tracheotomy. *J Laryngol Otol* 1996; **110**: 723–6

4　Brasavola AM. Libris de Ratione Victus in Morbis Acutis, Hippocratis et Galenii Commentaria et Annotationes. Pars IV, Scotum, Venetiis, 1546; 97–104

5　Morens DM. Death of a president. *New Engl J Med* 1999; **341(24)**: 1845–9

6　Jackson C. Tracheotomy. *Laryngoscope* 1909; **19**: 285–90

7　Lassen HCA. A preliminary report on the 1952 epidemic of poliomyelitis in Copenhagen with special reference to the treatment of respiratory insufficiency. *Lancet* 1953; **1**: 37–41

8　Commentaria in Primam fen Primi Libri Canonis Avicennae. Iacobum Sarcinam, Venetiis, 1626; 507–12

9　Shelden CH, Pudenz RH, Freshwater DB, Crue BL. A new method for tracheostomy. *J Neurosurg* 1955; **12**: 428–31

10　Toye FJ, Weinstein JD. A percutaneous tracheostomy device. *Surgery* 1969; **65**: 384–9

11　Brantigan CO, Grow Sr JB. Cricothyroidotomy: elective use in respiratory problems requiring tracheotomy. *J Thorac Cardiovasc Surg* 1976; **71**: 72–81

12　Ciaglia P, Firsching R, Syniec C. Elective Percutaneous Dilatational Tracheostomy. *Chest* 1985; **87**: 715–9

13　Bodenham A, Diament R, Cohen A, Webster N. Percutaneous dilational tracheostomy. A bedside procedure on the intensive care unit. *Anaesthesia* 1991; **46**: 570–2

14　Schachner A, Ovil Y, Sidi J, Rogev M, Helibronn Y, Levy MJ. Percutaneous tracheostomy – a new method. *Crit Care Med* 1989; **17**: 1052–6

15　Whittet HB, Marks N, Waldmann C, Douglas S. The 'Percutrac': a minimally invasive percutaneous tracheostomy device. *Minimal Invas Ther* 1993; **2**: 319–24

16　Griggs WM, Worthley LI, Gilligan JE, Thomas PD, Myburg JA. A simple percutaneous tracheostomy technique. *Surg Gynecol Obstet* 1990; **170**: 543–5

17　Fantoni A, Ripamonti D. A non-derivative, non-surgical tracheostomy: the translaryngeal method. *Intens Care Med* 1997; **23**: 386–92

18　Bewsher MS, Adams AM, Clarke CWM, McConachie I, Kelly DR. Evaluation of a new percutaneous dilatational tracheostomy set. *Anaesthesia* 2001; **56**: 859–64

19　Frova G, Quintel M. A new simple method for percutaneous tracheostomy: controlled rotating dilation. *Intens Care Med* 2002; **28**: 299–303

20 Mathews HR, Hopkinson RB. Treatment of sputum retention by minitracheotomy. *Br J Surg* 1984; **71**: 147–50

21 Corke C, Cranswick P. A Seldinger technique for minitracheostomy insertion. *Anaesth Intens Care* 1988; **16**: 206–7

22 Paw HGW, Turner S. The current state of percutaneous tracheostomy in intensive care: a postal survey. *Clin Intens Care* 2002; **13**: 95–101

23 Cooper RM. Use and safety of percutaneous tracheostomy in intensive care. *Anaesthesia* 1998; **53**: 1209–27

2 Anatomy of the Trachea

Basic anatomy

The trachea (Figures 2.1 and 2.2) begins at the level of the C6 vertebra in continuity with the larynx, being attached to the lower margin of the cricoid cartilage by the cricotracheal ligament. The trachea is a mobile cartilaginous and membranous tube made up of 16–20 C-shaped rings of hyaline cartilage, which provide rigidity and maintain the patency of the tube. Posteriorly, the circumference is flattened slightly by the presence of the fibroelastic membrane stretching between the ends of each cartilaginous ring. The membrane has smooth muscle embedded in it. This muscle has been called the trachealis muscle and is involved in regulating the diameter of the trachea. The trachea begins at the lower end of the cricoid cartilage and extends downwards in the midline of the neck to the carina. In an adult, the traches is 10–12 cm long and 2.5 cm in diameter, but this varies with age, sex and race. Individuals with a short stature tend to have smaller tracheas. The root of the index finger gives a rough estimation of tracheal diameter. It is a unique structure in the body and to date, no natural or prosthetic material has been found satisfactory for reconstructive surgery. This is one reason why stenotic or other complications of the trachea are so feared by medical practitioners.

In the elderly or diseased patient, the trachea may become considerably distorted and have significant acute angulations (Figures 2.3 and 2.4). Any change in the angle of the cervical or upper thoracic spine will cause similar angulation of the trachea.[1]

In the neck, the trachea is located relatively close to the anterior skin surface and, as it descends into the thoracic cavity, it moves posteriorly (Figure 2.5). This backward angulation in relation to skin

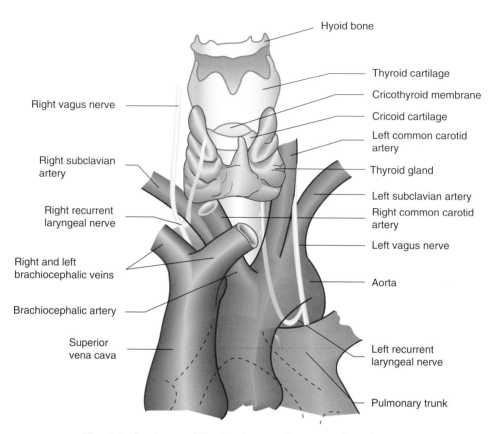

Fig. 2.1 **Anatomy of the trachea and surrounding tissues. (Redrawn from Grillo HC (Ed).** *Surgery of the Trachea and Bronchi*. **2004: BC Decker Inc; Hamilton, Ontario.)**

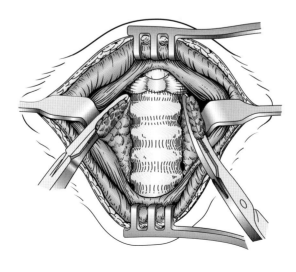

Fig. 2.2 **Surgical dissection for open thyroidectomy: clamps are applied to divided thyroid isthmus.**

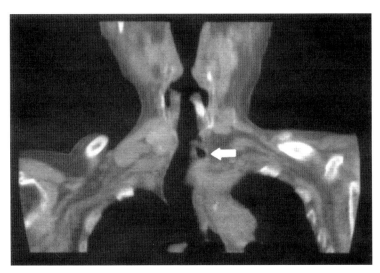

Fig. 2.3 CT of the neck showing a tracheal diverticulum about 2 cm below vocal cords (white arrow). Reproduced with permission.[1]

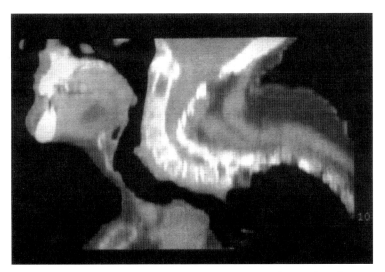

Fig. 2.4 CT showing a 90° bend in the subglottic trachea because of pronounced cervical lordosis secondary to a thoracic kyphosis. Reproduced with permission.[1]

on the neck or the sternum may be more pronounced in the elderly patient with chronic lung disease or collapsed vertebrae.

In the normal anatomic position, approximately 50% of the trachea (5 cm) is in the thoracic cavity and 50% is above the thoracic inlet. The position of the trachea is markedly affected by whether the neck

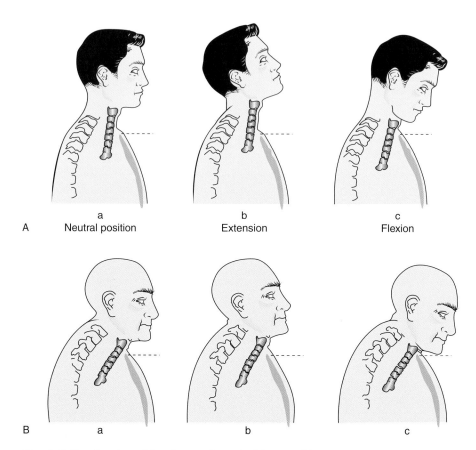

A   a   Neutral position   b   Extension   c   Flexion

B   a   b   c

Fig. 2.5 Tracheal position in youth and old age with cervical extension and flexion. The trachea is much more vertical on lateral projection in youth (A) than in old age (B). A, (a) In youth, approximately one-third of the trachea is in the neck above the sternum (*dashed line*) in neutral position. (b) With cervical extension, one-half or more rises into the neck. (c) Most of the trachea devolves into the thorax on full flexion. B, In the aged, the level of the larynx (a) changes little with attempted cervical (b) extension and (c) flexion. Surgical implications are obvious. (Redrawn with permission from Grillo HC (Ed) *Surgery of the Trachea and Bronchi*. 2004: BC Decker Inc; Hamilton, Ontario.)

is flexed or extended (Figure 2.5). With the neck in extension, a larger portion of the trachea becomes extra-thoracic. This has implications for the positioning of the skin incision and tracheal stoma, which will move in relation to each other in the neck. Care should therefore be taken to avoid extremes of extension during tracheostomy, as on assuming a more neutral position, the tracheal stoma may come to lie behind the sternum (see Chapter 13: Tips and Tricks). Equally, in the patient with a short, fat neck, it may be impossible to access lower tracheal rings unless the tracheal stoma is retrosternal. The latter should be avoided due to potential difficulties in changing tubes and the close proximity of the great vessels.

Anatomical relations and blood supply

In the neck, the anterior surface of the trachea is covered by the isthmus of the thyroid, the inferior thyroid veins, the thyroidea ima artery, the sternothyroid and sternohyoid muscles, cervical fascia, and the anastomosing branches of the anterior jugular veins. Skin, platysma, fascia, sternocleidomastoid and strap muscles (sternohyoid, omohyoid and sternothyroid) lie superficially. Laterally, the upper trachea is covered by the lobes of the thyroid gland, and the contents of the carotid sheath (carotid arteries, internal jugular vein, vagus nerve and ansa cervicalis). The recurrent laryngeal nerves run in the tracheoesophageal groove. In the neck, the posterior fibroelastic membranous wall of the trachea abuts the oesophagus, which is vulnerable if the posterior tracheal wall is damaged. As the trachea descends into the upper thoracic cavity, it is surrounded by many vital structures. At the level of the thoracic inlet, immediately to the right of the trachea, lies the innominate artery and anteriorly, the left innominate vein. The location of the innominate (brachiocephalic) vessels is important, as a tracheostomy placed too low in the trachea may cause the tube to erode into such vessels and produce massive haemorrhage from a tracheoinnominate fistula.

The anterior jugular vein begins just below the chin, by the union of several small veins. It lies superficially and runs down the neck very close to the midline on either side, crossing the thyroid isthmus (Figure 2.6). Just above the suprasternal notch, the veins of the two sides are united by a transverse trunk called the jugular arch. The vein then turns sharply laterally and passes deep to the sternocleidomastoid muscle to drain into the external jugular vein. The course of such veins is very variable. Such veins may become very large in the presence of tricuspid regurgitation or as a result of collateral venous flow in the presence of a thrombosed jugular or subclavian vein.

Following surgery to the neck, vessels may become adherent to the trachea placing them at risk during tracheostomy procedures. In

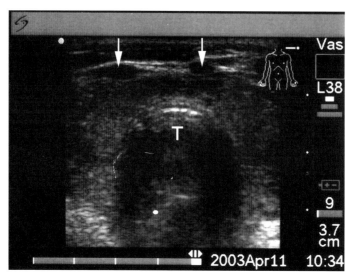

Fig. 2.6 Anterior jugular veins (arrows) in front of the trachea (T).

addition, in the elderly with ectatic or diseased vessels, the subclavian artery may arise up into the neck (see Chapter 11: Complications of Percutaneous Tracheostomy).

The isthmus of the thyroid gland lies in front of the second, third and fourth rings of the trachea. In some patients (>50% of population), a pyramidal lobe projects upwards from the isthmus, generally to the left of the midline (Figure 2.7). It may be attached to the inferior border of the hyoid bone by the levator glandulae thyroideae, a fibromuscular tissue. The inferior thyroid veins lie in front of the fifth, sixth and seventh rings of the trachea. The inferior thyroid veins of the two sides anastomose with one another as they descend in front of the trachea and drain into the left brachiocephalic vein in the thorax. The thyroidea ima artery, when present, ascends in front of the trachea to enter the lower part of the isthmus in 3% of the population. It can arise from the brachiocephalic trunk, arch of the aorta or right common carotid artery.

The blood supply to the cervical trachea is primarily from the inferior thyroid artery. The artery runs behind the common carotid artery and, in the most common pattern, sends three branches to the upper trachea. Disruption to such vessels during thyroidectomy may be one

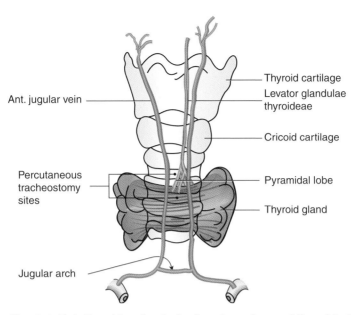

Fig. 2.7 Relationship of anterior jugular veins and thyroid gland to the trachea.

cause of tracheomalacia. The arterial supply to the thoracic trachea is more variable and comes from a combination of vessels from either the innominate or the subclavian arteries. These branches approach the trachea laterally and then anastomose to form a longitudinal vessel that gives off segmental branches to supply the trachea. The arterial supply of the tracheal mucosa comes from a rich plexus of vessels. Anteriorly and laterally, the plexus is supplied by small 'twigs' arising from the intercartilaginous branches. Posteriorly, the plexus is supplied by the 'twigs' from oesophageal vessels. The cartilaginous rings of the trachea do not have a specific blood supply; rather they receive their nutrition via diffusion of nutrients from the submucosal plexus. There is no external plexus to supply the cartilage, so when the inside of the trachea is compressed for long periods of time, such as from the cuff of an overinflated endotracheal tube or tracheostomy tube, the cartilage becomes ischaemic, and this can lead to scarring and tracheal stenosis. Equally, if the mucosa is damaged during the percutaneous tracheostomy procedures, similar problems may ensue. The blood supply to the mucosa is vulnerable to excessive cuff pressure and studies have shown that inflation pressures above 30 cm H_2O (22 mmHg) will produce ischaemia.[2]

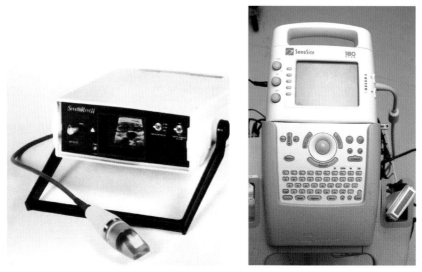

Fig. 2.8 Examples of portable ultrasound probes.

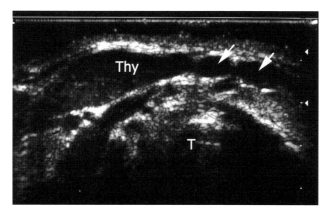

Fig. 2.9 Ultrasound image showing two large midline anterior jugular veins (white arrows) and the thyroid gland (Thy) in front of the trachea (T).

It has always been assumed that the midline is avascular and if a tracheostomy is situated in the midline, bleeding is unlikely. This assumption is not always true. Ultrasound probes are useful to visualise such vessels (Figure 2.8). An ultrasound image of the neck of one of the authors' (Henry G.W. Paw) clearly shows two anterior neck veins in the midline (Figure 2.9).

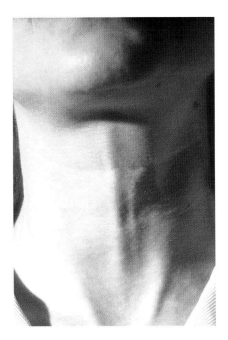

Fig. 2.10 Prominent midline anterior jugular vein, whilst performing a Valsalva manoeuvre.

With the routine use of ultrasound prior to performing a percutaneous tracheostomy, the authors have found that it is not uncommon to have veins running down the midline (Figure 2.10).

Innervation

Superficially, the sensory innervation of skin overlying the trachea is from the cervical plexus (roots C2, 3, 4). This can be blocked by infiltration of local anaesthetic or a bilateral superficial cervical plexus block, where the nerve curls round the posterior border of sternomastoid muscle. The sensory innervation of the trachea and vocal cords is supplied by the vagus nerves via the recurrent laryngeal nerves. This can be blocked by injection of local anaesthetic through the cricothyroid membrane or direct instillation down a tracheal tube or bronchoscope.

References

1 Davies R. Difficult tracheal intubation secondary to a tracheal diverticulum and a 90 degree deviation in the trachea. *Anaesthesia* 2000; **55**: 923–5

2   Seegobin RD, van Hasselt GL. Endotracheal cuff pressure and tracheal mucosal blood flow: endoscopic study of effects of four large volume cuffs. *Br Med J* 1984; **228**: 965–8

Further reading

Allen MS. Surgical anatomy of the trachea. *Chest Surg Clin North Am* 1996; **6**: 627–35

Sinnatamby CS. *Last's Anatomy Regional and Applied*, 10th edition. Churchill Livingstone, 1999

Grillo HC. Anatomy of the trachea 39–59 in Grillo HC. Ed. *Surgery of the Trachea and Bronchi* 2004 BC Decker, Hamilton, Ontario

3 Indications and Timing of Tracheostomy

An artificial airway is used in patients requiring intensive care to facilitate assisted ventilation, administration of high FiO_2, removal of respiratory secretions and to protect the airway from aspiration. Initially, this is usually most conveniently provided by translaryngeal intubation via the nose or mouth. Translaryngeal intubation has the advantage of speed and convenience in the initial phase. However, the patient usually requires an anaesthetic to allow laryngoscopy and tracheal intubation. Following translaryngeal intubation, significant quantities of sedative and analgesic drugs are required to tolerate the ET tube.

By contrast, a tracheostomy tube, even though it requires a surgical incision for insertion, is much more comfortable for the patient. Typically, within a few hours following insertion, the patient will be able to tolerate the tracheostomy tube without significant doses of sedative or analgesic drugs. There is usually a marked reduction in the requirement for such drugs following conversion of translaryngeal intubation to tracheostomy. This is probably best explained by reference to the reduction in the density of sensory and motor innervation, on descent from the nose, mouth and tongue, down into the larynx. This is diagrammatically represented in the so-called 'homunculus' (Figure 3.1). Similar observations have been made in the past when the comfort of pharyngostomy feeding tube placement was compared to tubes passed through the nose or mouth.

Tracheostomy may be necessary in upper airway obstruction caused by trauma, infection, malignancy, laryngeal or subcricoid stenosis, and bilateral recurrent laryngeal nerve palsy. Emergency upper airway obstruction is a relative contraindication for percutaneous tracheostomy due to uncertainties as to the site of obstruction. The classical cited

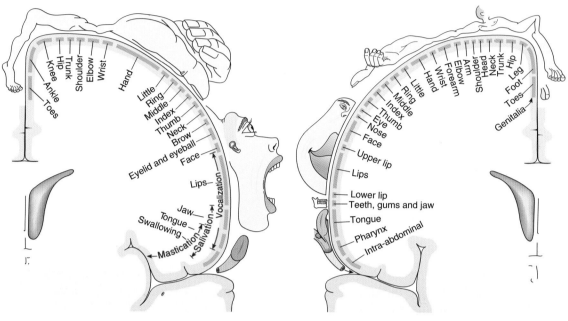

Fig. 3.1 **Homunculus.**

example is that of the laryngeal tumour extending a variable distance down into the trachea with the potential for loss of the airway. In patients with laryngeal incompetence (e.g. after cerebrovascular accident), a tracheostomy may also be useful to prevent aspiration and aid clearance of secretions. The indications for tracheostomy are listed in Box 3.1.

There has been some discussion in the past as to whether patients who are likely to require long-term tracheostomy placement should have an open surgical placement in the belief that tube changes are easier after open *versus* percutaneous techniques. There is little evidence for such beliefs except perhaps in the first week following percutaneous placement, when tracts are relatively tight around the tube. Careful consideration should, however, be given to the choice of tube and other aspects of airway management.[1]

There is also a place for percutaneous tracheostomy in ward-based patients who may never have been on an intensive care unit. Such

Box 3.1 Indications for tracheostomy in the critically ill

- Patient comfort
- Aid to weaning
- Failed extubation
- Long-term ventilation
- Sputum retention
- Inadequate cough
- End stage respiratory disease
- Severe neuromuscular weakness
- Significant brain injury
- Upper airway obstruction
- Laryngeal incompetence/damage

procedures may be performed on ward patients with respiratory failure or inadequate cough from many different causes, in the hope that the need for assisted ventilation or ICU admission can be avoided. Patients can be brought up to an anaesthetic room or operating theatre for such procedures under a brief general anaesthetic. The airway is secured by ET intubation and the lungs are re-expanded by positive pressure ventilation and removal of tracheal secretions, prior to the procedure. Procedures can be performed under local anaesthesia but it is not pleasant for the patient. Even when adequate local anaesthesia is achieved, the forces used for dilation are uncomfortable.

Traditionally, there has been a reluctance to perform early tracheostomy and patients have undergone repeated trials of extubation and re-intubation prior to eventually proceeding to a tracheostomy for weaning. They therefore ran the risk of developing complications both from prolonged translaryngeal intubation (Box 3.2) and the subsequent tracheostomy. We believe we should try to reduce the risks of this 'double insult'.

Patients who can be identified as being very likely to require a tracheostomy for weaning (Box 3.3), should have a tracheostomy procedure sooner rather than later to reduce the complications of prolonged translaryngeal intubation (Figures 3.2–3.5).

Box 3.2 **Complications of prolonged translaryngeal intubation**

- Side effects of sedative and analgesic drugs
- Difficulties in mouth care
- Difficulties in swallowing
- Immobility
- Nasal erosions
- Nasal sinusitis
- Sore mouth
- Communication difficulties
- Laryngeal damage
- Subglottic stenosis
- Difficulties with tube changes
- Trauma from repeated extubation/re-intubation sequences

Box 3.3 **Indications for consideration of early tracheostomy**

- Severe brain injury
- High spinal cord injury
- Severe neuromuscular disease, e.g. Guillain Barré syndrome
- Severe pancreatitis with open abdomen
- Limited cardiorespiratory reserve
- Morbid obesity
- Obstructive sleep apnoea
- Bulbar palsy
- Severe underlying medical disorders

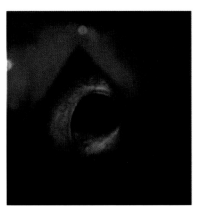

Fig. 3.2 Subglottic stenosis following prolonged oral ET intubation.

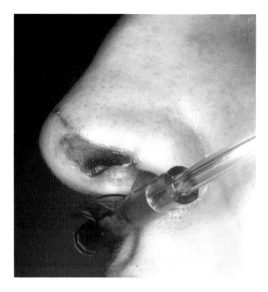

Fig. 3.3 Skin erosion of the nose following nasal ET intubation in a young girl.

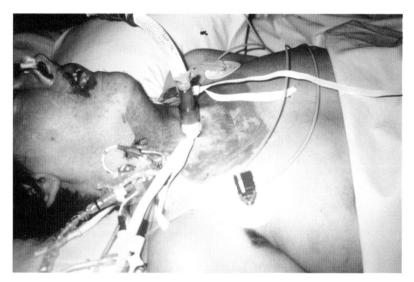

Fig. 3.4 Percutaneous tracheostomy performed in a patient with ulcerated mouth and lips (mechanical damage plus herpes infection) following prolonged oral ET intubation.

Timing

On the ICU, increasing patient comfort is one of the most common reasons for performing a tracheostomy. It reduces the need for sedation and in most cases no sedation is required at all. This facilitates

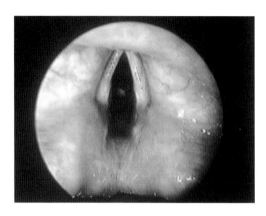

Fig. 3.5 Erosions to posterior aspect of glottis following prolonged ET intubation (percutaneous tracheostomy *in situ*).

earlier weaning from the ventilator. Compared to translaryngeal intubation, airway resistance, dead space and the work of breathing are reduced, which will further aid the process of weaning.

In some patients, it is difficult to predict who will be successfully weaned. In such a situation, one or more trials of extubation may be used as part of the weaning strategy. Repeated failures of extubation suggest that the patient requires prolonged tracheal intubation with or without assisted ventilation and is one indication for tracheostomy. Other cases can be anticipated to require prolonged tracheal intubation and assisted ventilation (Box 3.3), including patients with severe pre-existing COPD and weakness from Guillain Barré syndrome or critical illness polyneuropathy.

Despite the perceived advantages of tracheostomy in these scenarios, there is no consensus as to when a tracheostomy should be performed.[2] Traditionally, tracheostomy was considered after about 10 days of assisted ventilation. Increasingly earlier tracheostomies (as early as within 2 days of translaryngeal intubation) are now performed. The popularity of percutaneous tracheostomy has resulted in an increased proportion of ICU patients undergoing tracheostomy earlier.[3] It has been suggested that early tracheostomy may shorten the length of ICU stay and decreases the incidence of nosocomial pneumonias. However, it is also possible that more tracheostomies are being performed than is necessary. Some patients may be able to avoid tracheostomy if further time is allowed to improve their general condition and respiratory function. The timing should be individualised in each case. In patients with sputum

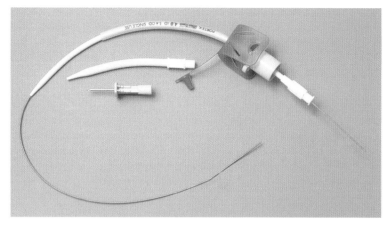

Fig. 3.6 Mini-Trach II – Seldinger, ID 4 mm (SIMS Portex).

retention, a small-bore cricothyroidotomy tube, such as the Mini-Trach II (Figure 3.6) may be worth considering before deciding on a formal larger-bore tracheostomy.

There are no definitive studies showing improved weaning or outcome with percutaneous tracheostomy when compared with translaryngeal intubation. Such studies are still required, particularly if the number of percutaneous tracheostomy procedures is to continue to increase. However, many centres would be reluctant to go back to delaying procedures for the length of time required to show a difference in such trials. Any trial would need large numbers and is likely to require external funding to support recruitment and organisation of multiple centres. Those studies that have started in this area have tended to finish prematurely due to recruitment difficulties.[4,5] The UK Intensive care society (ICS) has plans to perform a large randomised controlled study of early versus late tracheostomy in patients requiring intensive care in 2004. This study is being organised by Dr Duncan Young (John Radcliffe Hospital Oxford). The detailed protocol can be accessed on the ICS website www.ics.ac.uk.

References

1   Heffner JE. Tracheostomy management in the chronically ventilated patient. *Clin Chest Med* 2001; **22**: 55–69
2   Heffner JE. Tracheotomy application and timing. *Clin Chest Med* 2003; **24**: 389–98

3   Simpson TP, Day CJE, Jewkes CF, Manara AR. The impact of percutaneous tracheostomy on intensive care unit practice and training. *Anaesthesia* 1999; **54**: 186–9

4   Kluger Y, *et al*. Early tracheostomy in trauma patients. *Eur J Emerg Med* 1996; **3**: 95–101

5   Rodriguez JL, *et al*. Early tracheostomy for primary airway management in the surgical critical care setting. *Surgery* 1990; **108**: 655–9

Further reading

Benjamin B. Laryngeal Trauma from Intubation: Endoscopic Evaluation and Classification. 2013–35 in Charles W Cummings *et al*. (Eds). *Otolaryngology Head and Neck Surgery*, 3rd edition. Volume 3: 1998 Mosby, London

4 Contraindications to Tracheostomy

The list of situations where percutaneous tracheostomy is absolutely contraindicated (Box 4.1) has shrunk with increasing experience of the users and the availability of fibreoptic bronchoscopy and ultrasound imaging.

Box 4.1 Absolute contraindications to percutaneous tracheostomy

- Unstable cervical spinal fracture
- Children <12 years old
- Uncorrectable coagulopathy
- Local infection
- Local malignancy

Contraindications to percutaneous tracheostomy are relative (Box 4.2) and are dependent on the skill and confidence of the operator. One of the authors (Andrew R. Bodenham) believes that there are few situations where percutaneous tracheostomy is absolutely contraindicated if a tracheostomy is required for other clinical indications. He has performed the procedure on patients with local malignancy and spinal injury. Decisions should be individualised for each patient.

Analysis of clinical trials comparing at least two percutaneous tracheostomy techniques did not suggest significant differences in terms of overall complications.[1] Because each technique has its own unique features, one particular technique may be more suitable in patients with certain contraindications. Percutaneous tracheostomy is

---

Box 4.2 Relative contraindications to percutaneous tracheostomy

- Large goitre
- Emergency airway access
- Morbid obesity
- Adolescent >12 years old
- Tracheomalacia
- FiO_2 requirement >0.6
- Cardiovascular instability
- Significant coagulopathy/thrombocytopenia
- Previous tracheostomy
- Previous neck surgery/radiotherapy
- Surgical wounds next to the tracheostomy site
- Anatomical or other abnormalities in the neck
- Extensive burns to the neck
- Patient unlikely to survive >48 h

---

not normally performed on children under 16 years of age due to their highly elastic and easily collapsible tracheas. The translaryngeal (Fantoni) technique is theoretically feasible in older children or young adults, as the technique does not require anteroposterior pressure.

The prevalence of morbidly obese patients is increasing in the developed countries. Many clinicians still consider morbid obesity a contraindication for percutaneous tracheostomy because of unfavourable neck anatomy and an increased complication rate. With experience, and the use of fibreoptic bronchoscopy and ultrasound imaging, it is possible to perform percutaneous tracheostomy in morbidly obese patients and patients who have had previous tracheostomy. Indeed, it may be preferable in these patients to perform the tracheostomy percutaneously rather than with an open surgical technique. One of the authors (Henry G.W. Paw) now routinely scans the neck with ultrasound before performing a percutaneous tracheostomy. As a result of being able to see the anatomy, many cases that would previously have been referred for open surgical tracheostomy have been successfully performed percutaneously (Figure 4.1).

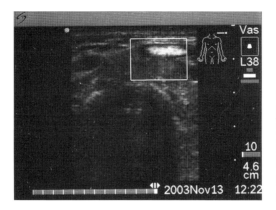

Fig. 4.1 Large 1.5 cm anterior jugular vein very close to the midline highlighted using Doppler imaging (white box). Percutaneous tracheostomy was successfully inserted just off centre (avoiding the vein).

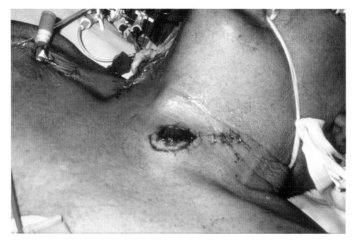

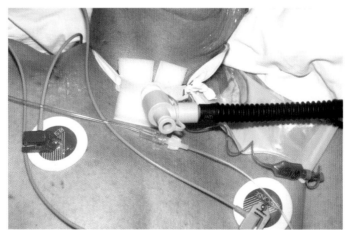

Fig. 4.2 Two different patients with previous neck surgery (defunctioning of cervical oesophagus in both cases), before and after percutaneous tracheostomy. The tracheostomy incision was kept as small as possible and positioned to one side of the midline to ensure separation of the two wounds.

In other cases, the small incision and minimal tissue dissection associated with percutaneous tracheostomy allows tracheostomy to be safely performed alongside other pathology or surgical interventions in the neck (Figure 4.2).

In the past, tracheostomy was often delayed in patients who had undergone previous median sternotomy. The assumption was that the close proximity of the sternal wound and tracheostomy lead to contamination of the sternotomy with micro-organisms from the airway, resulting in sternal infection or mediastinitis.[2] The fear of perioperative mediastinitis still leads many clinicians to be hesitant about performing a tracheostomy within the first two post-operative weeks.[3] This fear may be based on several studies showing an increase risk of tracheostomy wound infection after open surgical tracheostomy.[4] Purulent secretions from the tracheostomy are a cause of concern, particularly in close proximity to sternal or cervical wounds (e.g. after oesophageal surgery). Stoma infection is uncommon with percutaneous tracheostomy. In patients with fresh surgical wounds close to the tracheostomy site, the percutaneous technique is not necessarily a contraindication.

The most common complication using the forceps-based techniques (Grigg's) is moderate bleeding in patients with normal coagulation. It is therefore not advisable to perform percutaneous tracheostomy using the Grigg's technique in patients with a coagulopathy or thrombocytopenia. The translaryngeal technique (Fantoni's) may be preferable in patients at increased risk of bleeding, because stoma dilatation is achieved with the tracheostomy cannula itself. Achieving dilatation to the exact degree required results in the cannula fitting snugly, thereby exerting pressure on the wound edges and reducing bleeding. This technique has been successfully used in a severely haemophiliac patient who had inhibitors to factor XIII.[5]

Emergency use of percutaneous tracheostomy

Traditional teaching has suggested that percutaneous techniques for tracheostomy should be reserved for the elective situation. The origin of these arguments can be debated but they do not readily stand scrutiny. Percutaneous techniques are generally much quicker than open surgical procedures, particularly in the absence of a skilled ENT, thoracic or head and neck surgeon who is used to dealing with such procedures on a regular basis. Most medical or surgical personnel attending emergency situations do not have such skills.

There is now a generation of anaesthetists and intensivists who have extensive experience of percutaneous tracheostomy. It is inevitable that such techniques are likely to be used if translaryngeal intubation proves impossible. Such individuals rarely have any skilled practice in open procedures. It is likely that experience gained on intensive care units may provide a valuable opportunity for anaesthetists and others to gain such experience in a real patient situation. Previous experience in percutaneous tracheostomy is likely to increase the chances of a successful outcome with tubes placed via an emergency cricothyroidotomy or tracheostomy using open or percutaneous techniques. The ability to pass guidewires quickly and effectively into the trachea gives the opportunity for practitioners to use other airway techniques such as retrograde intubation, again improving their skills in the emergency situation.

References

1   Byhahn C. A useful and safe intervention: current techniques of percutaneous tracheostomy. *Int J Intens Care* 2003; **10**: 155–65
2   Brown AH, *et al*. The complications of median sternotomy. *J Thorac Cardiovasc Surg* 1969; **58**: 189–97
3   Hübner N, *et al*. Percutaneous dilatational tracheostomy done early after cardiac surgery: outcome and incidence of mediastinitis. *Thorac Cardiovasc Surg* 1998; **46**: 89–92
4   Freeman BD, *et al*. A meta-analysis of prospective trials comparing percutaneous and surgical tracheostomy in critically ill patients. *Chest* 2000; **118**: 1412–8
5   Byhahn C, Lischke V, Westphal K. Translaryngeal tracheostomy in highly unstable patients. *Anaesthesia* 2000; **55**: 678–82

5 Advantages of Tracheostomy *versus* Translaryngeal Intubation

Prolonged assisted ventilation using translaryngeal nasal or orotracheal tubes is associated with a number of problems. Translaryngeal tracheal tubes are uncomfortable and often require the patient to be heavily sedated, which has its own inherent problems. Orotracheal tubes are generally more uncomfortable than nasal tubes. Tracheostomy is better tolerated (Figure 5.1), when compared with both nasal and orotracheal intubations. One explanation for this observation is the reduction in neuronal innervation on descending from the face to the neck. This is illustrated in the so-called 'homunculus' (Figure 5.2). After a few hours of tracheostomy tube placement, patients often do not require any further sedative or analgesic agent in order to tolerate the tube. Similar findings have been noted when feeding tubes are placed by a pharyngostomy compared to the nasal route.[2]

Translaryngeal tracheal tubes are more liable to occlusion by the patient biting on the tube, kinking or build up of secretions. The length and contours of a tracheal tube make it more difficult to pass catheters for effective tracheobronchial suctioning of secretions.

Oral tubes can be difficult to secure and constant movements increase the chance of tracheal mucosa damage. They also prevent adequate oral hygiene procedures and may lead to a very sore mouth and lips.

Nasal tubes are easier to secure, less liable to occlusion and more comfortable than oral tracheal tubes, but they require a smaller-bore tube and are associated with infections in the paranasal sinuses in adults (Figure 5.3) or nasal erosions (Figure 5.4). Their use is

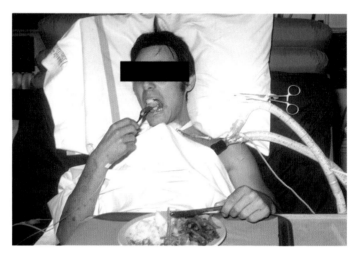

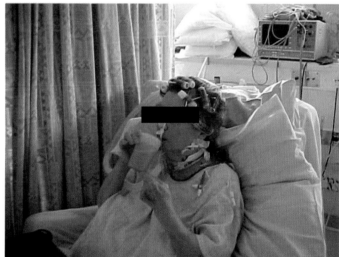

Fig. 5.1 Two ventilator-dependent patients recovering from severe meningococcal sepsis and an infective exacerbation of severe COPD, respectively. Such oral nutrition and mobilisation would have been difficult to achieve with a translaryngeal tube (reproduced with patients' permission).

relatively contraindicated in the presence of a coagulopathy. A tracheostomy can reduce or eliminate these problems.

Effective verbal communication may be possible in the patient with a tracheostomy, either by deflation of the cuff or the use of a fenestrated (speaking) tracheostomy tube, which allows expired gas to pass upwards through the vocal cords. There are a number of different

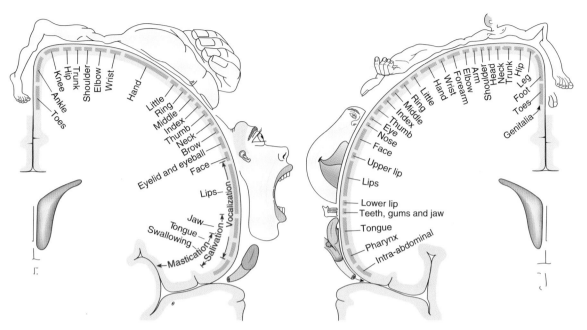

Fig. 5.2 Homunculus (Greek 'little man'): below the larynx there is very little representation in both motor and sensory pathways. This is represented by the visual size of the image. Note the very large size of lips, nose and tongue, reflecting the very rich innervation of these structures.

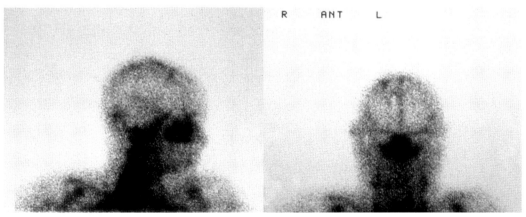

Fig. 5.3 Adult male patient shows take up of radioactive labelled white cells in paranasal sinuses, lateral (left) and anterior posterior (right) views, following prolonged nasotracheal intubation.

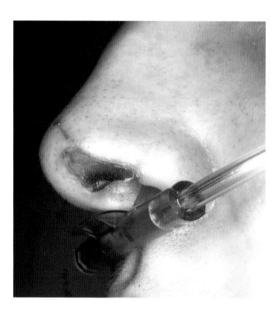

Fig. 5.4 Nasal erosion following nasotracheal intubation.

valves designed to redirect expiratory gas up through the vocal cords to allow speech. Other tubes have an additional small-bore channel to direct pressurised air or oxygen upwards from below the vocal cords (see Chapter 8: Tracheostomy Tubes, page 69).

Tracheostomy reduces the upper airway anatomical dead space by up to 150 ml or 50%. The shorter length and shape of the tracheostomy tube also reduces its resistance to airflow. This benefits the patient, with limited respiratory reserve, by reducing the work of breathing when compared to translaryngeal tracheal tubes. The reduced work of breathing may reduce fatigue and reduce the time the patient remains ventilator dependent.

Seamless transitions between different modes of respiratory support during weaning are easy with a tracheostomy *in situ*. There is no need for repeated trials of extubation, and if this then fails, subsequent anaesthesia and re-intubation. Further accumulation of sedative and analgesic drugs and potential trauma to the larynx and trachea are avoided.

It is common for patients in the recovery phase of critical illness to have adequate respiratory function to breath unaided, but not to clear respiratory secretions. Tracheostomy allows avoidance of assisted ventilation or accelerated weaning from it, whilst tracheal secretions are controlled. Many patients can be discharged whilst still ventilator/CPAP/suction-dependent to lower dependency areas. Trials to prove such benefits are difficult to perform in this population of patients, and positive results that prove the case for tracheostomy have been elusive, but the advantages of tracheostomy over nasal or orotracheal intubation are summarised in Box 5.1.

Box 5.1 Potential advantages of tracheostomy

- Increased patient comfort
- Increased tolerance of assisted ventilation
- Reduced sedation/analgesia
- More effective tracheobronchial suctioning of secretions
- Encourages oral nutrition
- Reduced risk of accidental extubation
- Facilitates mouth care
- Verbal communication possible
- Decreased dead space
- Reduced work of breathing
- Easier mobilisation
- Tubes can be changed without sedative drugs and laryngoscopy
- Earlier weaning from assisted ventilation
- Earlier discharge from critical care unit

Clinicians should be aware of what is called the 'double insult': i.e. the risks of both a prolonged period of translaryngeal intubation (Box 5.2)

Box 5.2 Disadvantages of translaryngeal intubation

- Requires significant use of sedative analgesics to tolerate the tube
- Nasal sinusitis
- Minor damage to laryngeal structures is common
- Occasional severe long-term damage to larynx/trachea
- Swallowing difficulty
- Communication difficulties
- Requires skilled personnel, anaesthesia and muscle relaxants to intubate/re-intubate
- Double insult if prolonged then converted to tracheostomy

> **Box 5.3 Disadvantages of tracheostomy**
>
> - Invasive traumatic procedure with occasional severe long-term complications in the trachea or other structures
> - Early procedures may have been avoidable
> - The procedure takes time and resources to perform
> - Learning curve for operators

and subsequent tracheostomy (Box 5.3), in a patient whose condition is such that a subsequent tracheostomy is inevitable if they survive the early course of their illness. An early tracheostomy should be considered in such patients (see Chapter 3: Indications and Timing).

References

1 Penfield W, Rasmussen T. *The Cerebral Cortex in Man*. New York: Macmillan, 1950
2 du Plessis JJ. Percutaneous pharyngostomy versus gastric tube placement in head injured patients. A prospective comparative study of 50 patients. *Acta Neurochir* 1992; **119**: 94–6

6 Advantages of Percutaneous *versus* Open Surgical Tracheostomy

Percutaneous tracheostomy has become an established technique in intensive care units in the UK and worldwide.[1] It is preferred to open surgical tracheostomy in the vast majority of critically ill patients.[2] In general, studies comparing the two techniques have tended to favour percutaneous techniques as being the safer of the two. Operator experience, preference and aftercare considerations are, however, important factors to consider.

When compared with open surgical techniques, percutaneous tracheostomy is safer, with a lower incidence of some complications including bleeding, infection and possibly tracheal stenosis.[3,4] There is, however, potential for a higher risk of operative complications due to the relatively blind nature of the procedure and the forces required for dilator and tube insertion.

There are inherent difficulties in performing comparative trials of techniques, which cannot be 'blinded'. Percutaneous tracheostomy is still evolving, with many variations in technique and the development of additional aids to safer practice (e.g. bronchoscopy and ultrasound guidance). Many practitioners have been reluctant to return to open procedures for the sole purpose of undertaking trials. Competent operators will experience low complication rates with either technique, and very large studies would be required to obtain the statistical power to show overall superiority of one technique over another. There are also now so many different kits available on the market that it is increasingly unlikely that definitive, large, comparative trials of all devices will be performed.

Percutaneous tracheostomy can be performed at the bedside, avoiding the risks associated with moving the patients to theatre. It is therefore ideal for patients on an ICU. There is also no need to wait for a theatre 'slot' and for a surgeon to become available, as an intensivist or anaesthetist can perform the technique safely. A prospective, randomised, controlled trial to compare the safety and efficacy of percutaneous tracheostomy with open surgical tracheostomy[5] found that the time from randomisation until tracheostomy was performed was considerably shorter for the percutaneous tracheostomy group (28.5 ± 27.9 h *versus* 100.4 ± 95.0 h; $p < 0.001$). Percutaneous tracheostomy was also quicker to perform (8.2 ± 4.9 min *versus* 33.9 ± 14.0 min; $p < 0.0001$) and associated with a lower incidence of complications. There was no significant difference in intra-procedural complications between the groups but post-procedural complication rates were 12% for percutaneous tracheostomy and 41% for open surgical tracheostomy ($p = 0.008$).

Although each percutaneous tracheostomy kit costs between £120 and £140, it is still cost-effective when compared with the open technique, as it can be performed at the bedside with no requirement for theatre time and staff. Several studies have shown significant cost savings.[6,7]

Percutaneous tracheostomy also has a better cosmetic result (Figure 6.1), due to the lower incidence of post-operative stomal infections, the smaller skin incision, and less dissection of tissues. There may be a reduced incidence of tracheal stenosis due to preservation of tracheal cartilage, but this has never been proven by a large clinical trial.

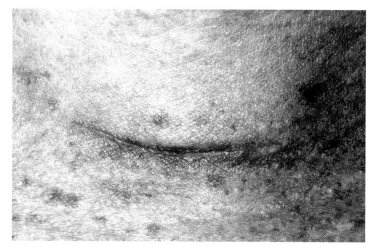

Fig. 6.1 **Scar following decannulation of percutaneous tracheostomy.**

The advantages of percutaneous tracheostomy over open surgical tracheostomy are summarised in Box 6.1.

> **Box 6.1 Advantages of percutaneous over open surgical tracheostomy**
>
> - Less risk of early significant bleeding
> - Reduced risk of stomal infection
> - Potentially lower incidence of tracheal stenosis
> - Can be performed more easily at the bedside
> - Avoid delays from unavailability of theatre session or surgeon
> - Minimal staff required
> - Open procedures often left to junior surgical trainees
> - Avoid risks of transferring patient to theatre
> - More cost-effective
> - Better cosmetic result
> - Quicker
> - Lower risk of tracheostomy tube dislodgement

Disadvantages of percutaneous tracheostomy

The disadvantages of percutaneous tracheostomy (Box 6.2) should also be appreciated, and the risks and benefits considered on an individual patient basis.

> **Box 6.2 Disadvantages of percutaneous over open surgical tracheostomy**
>
> - Occasional severe major bleed, tracheal rupture and oesophageal damage
> - Potential false passage (1–2% if bronchoscopy not used)
> - Can sometimes be difficult to replace dislodged cannula early after insertion
> - Reduced opportunities for learning surgical procedure
> - Ease of access allows occasional early unnecessary tracheostomy
> - Unproven in emergency situation
> - Safety in repeat tracheostomy procedures unproven
> - Safety in anatomical abnormalities uncertain
> - Kits not designed for longer stemmed tracheostomy tubes
> - Safety in children unclear

There is an inherent risk of tracheal damage and other complications related to insertion, with or without the use of bronchoscopy. Bronchoscopy should reduce, but does not eliminate, the risk of tracheal wall damage. During the insertion of the tracheostomy tube over the loading dilator, some anterior force has to be applied, which will result in a degree of tracheal collapse in the antero-posterior plane and an inability to visualise the actual insertion into the tracheal lumen. Posterior tracheal wall damage remains a disadvantage of techniques where instrumentation is passed from outside inwards.

Fantoni's translaryngeal technique, in which stomal dilation is achieved from inside the trachea to the outside with the tracheostomy cannula itself, is said to be safer with regards to posterior tracheal wall damage.[8] The new PercuTwist® set (Rüsch) with its screw-like threaded dilating device is also claimed to enhance safety. The anterior tracheal wall can be lifted during dilation, thus keeping the tracheal lumen open and enabling an unrestricted bronchoscopic view of the dilation site at any given time. There have not been large comparative studies to confirm clinical benefit from either technique.

Summary of complications (from some major publications)

Post-operative complications of percutaneous *versus* surgical tracheostomy

	PcT (%)	Surgical tracheostomy (%)
Bleeding	4.2	16.7
Stomal infection	4.2	33.3
Pneumothorax	4.2	4.2
Decannulation	12.5	45.8
Delayed healing	0	38
Tracheal stenosis	28	63
Cosmetic	9	25

Hazard P, Jones C, Benitone J. Comparative trial of standard operative tracheostomy with percutaneous tracheostomy. *Crit Care Med* 1991; **19**: 1018–24

Complications of percutaneous *versus* surgical tracheostomy

	PcT (%)	Surgical tracheostomy (%)
Intra-operative complications		
Paratracheal insertion	4	0
Transient hypotension	15	11
Transient hypoxia	0	11
Surgical emphysema	0	4
Minor bleeding	13	11
Loss of airway	0	4
Post-operative complications		
Accidental decannulation	4	15
Small bleed	4	11
Moderate bleed	0	0
Severe bleed	4	4
Wound/stomal infection	0	15

Friedman Y, *et al*. Comparison of percutaneous and surgical tracheostomies. *Chest* 1996; **110**: 480–5

References

1 Paw HGW, Turner S. The current state of percutaneous tracheostomy in intensive care: a postal survey. *Clin Intens Care* 2002; **13**: 95–101
2 Manara AR. Experience with percutaneous tracheostomy in intensive care: the procedure of choice? *Br J Oral Maxillofac Surg* 1994; **32**: 155–60
3 Lams E. Percutaneous and surgical tracheostomy. *Hospital Med* 2003; **64**: 36–39
4 Dulguerov P. Percutaneous or surgical tracheostomy; a meta analysis. *Crit Care Med* 1999; **27**: 1617–25
5 Friedman Y, *et al*. Comparison of percutaneous and surgical tracheostomies. *Chest* 1996; **110**: 480–5
6 Barba CA, *et al*. Bronchoscopic guidance makes percutaneous tracheostomy a safe, cost-effective and easy-to-teach procedure. *Surgery* 1995; **118**: 879–83
7 McHenry CR, Raeburn CD, Lange RL, Priebe PP. Percutaneous tracheostomy: a cost-effective alternative to standard open tracheostomy. *Am Surg* 1997; **63**: 646–52
8. Fantoni A, Ripamonti D. A non-derivative, non-surgical tracheostomy: the translaryngeal method. *Intens Care Med* 1977; **23**: 386–92

Different Techniques

Insertion of a tracheostomy tube at the bedside, using various commercial kits, has become a standard technique on many intensive care units. A number of different techniques have been established within the last few years, with or without the use of other aids like fibreoptic bronchoscopy.

The idea of inserting tracheostomy tubes into the trachea via a percutaneous as opposed to an open surgical technique is not new. Clearly what constitutes a percutaneous, as opposed to an open procedure, is open to debate. For many years, surgeons have tried to limit the size of incisions to reduce bleeding and surgical trauma to the patient. A skilled surgeon, operating in optimal circumstances, will be able to gain access to the trachea through a small incision with minimal disruption to surrounding tissues. Regrettably, the patient on the ICU does not usually offer such optimal conditions nor often benefit from the best local surgical expertise.

Historical devices have been limited by the risk of false passage and severe collateral damage. Instrumentation had to be sharp in order to enter the trachea with the obvious risk of damage to surrounding structures if misplaced. The advent of Seldinger techniques with flexible guidewires, plastic introducers and flexible tracheostomy tubes has revolutionised the success of such techniques. The majority of modern percutaneous tracheostomy kits are based on the concept of accessing the trachea with a needle and cannula. Needle position may be confirmed by aspiration of air from the trachea, capnography, aspiration of respiratory secretions or by direct vision with a bronchoscope. A guidewire can then be passed into the trachea and the tract dilated up with plastic dilators or forceps-based techniques. Once the tract is large enough, a tracheostomy tube can be passed into the trachea.

The safety of modern percutaneous techniques is reasonably well established when compared with traditional open surgical tracheostomy procedures. However, there have been few large controlled studies comparing one tracheostomy technique over another. Most have been performed by interested parties, either in the form of sponsored research by companies, or perhaps by the inventors of that particular tracheostomy technique. As such they cannot be considered truly independent sources for reference.

There is no doubt that experience is a key factor in making any technique safe and efficient. It is likely that the skill and experience of individual operators is more important than the particular design of one technique over another. All can be made to work. The true test comes when products are placed in the open market to be used by both expert and non-expert users. At the time of writing there is increasing concern about the proliferation of different airway devices, many of which have never been subjected to any sort of formal independent review.[1]

Long-term outcomes are also important. Follow-up studies are difficult, as there is a small overall risk of serious complications in skilled hands, high patient mortality and morbidity from other causes, in addition to imprecise definitions and identification of significant longer-term complications. Expensive, large, multicentre trials would be required, which interested parties would be unlikely to wish to sponsor. Kits and techniques are still developing and it can be argued that the optimum kit is yet to be marketed. Any studies need to be performed by the best operators for each technique at the top of their learning curve. Marketing strategies have limited the choice of kits in some countries, including the UK.

The use of the various kits in the UK is summarised in Table 7.1.[2] However, a more recent (2003) unpublished survey by Krishnan and colleagues in Leeds found that 97% of UK units performed PcT and the most popular kit was now the Blue Rhino Kit (62%), and use of the traditional Ciaglia kit had declined to 10%. Usage of other kits was similar in both surverys.

The usage of the various kits in the UK in 2002

Kit	Usage (%)
Cook Ciaglia sequential dilator kit	46.6
Cook Blue Rhino single-step dilator kit	31.3
Portex Griggs forceps dilator kit	17.3
Rüsch PercuQuick sequential dilator kit	3.3
Tyco Fantoni translaryngeal kit	1.3

Currently available kits for percutaneous tracheostomy

Technique	Characteristics	Manufacturers
Sequential dilators	Antegrade, multistep sequential dilatation with up to seven dilators	Cook Rüsch Portex
Dilating forceps	Antegrade, two-step dilatation with modified Howard-Kelly forceps	Portex Weiss
Fantoni's translaryngeal tracheostomy	Retrograde, single-step dilatation with the cannula itself	Tyco
Single-step dilator	Antegrade, single-step dilatation with a conically shaped dilator	Cook Portex
PercuTwist	Antegrade stoma formation with a self-tapping plastic screw	Rüsch

At the time of the survey, the new PercuTwist kit (Rüsch) was not available. All of the kits currently available for percutaneous tracheostomy are based on the Seldinger technique.[3] The trachea is punctured either blind or under bronchoscopic visualisation, and a guidewire is introduced into the tracheal lumen. The stoma is dilated in one or multiple steps in either an antegrade or retrograde direction to accommodate the tracheostomy tube. Table 7.2 provides a summary of the various kits currently available for percutaneous tracheostomy. The relative advantages and disadvantages of different methods of tracheal dilation are discussed in turn.

Plastic dilators

The most widely used techniques involve serial plastic dilators, as in kits manufactured by Cook (Figure 7.1) and Rüsch (Figure 7.2). Such

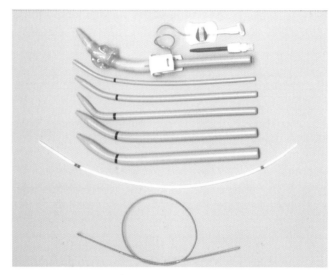

Fig. 7.1 Ciaglia sequential dilator kit (Cook).

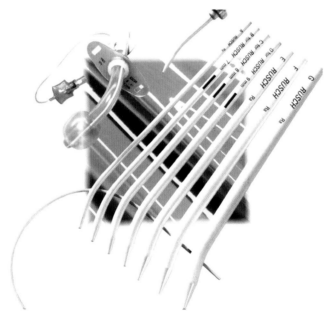

Fig. 7.2 PercuQuick sequential dilator kit (Rüsch).

dilators require considerable inward force to dilate up the tracheal wall and associated structures. As such, they have been associated with posterior tracheal wall tears and fracture of the tracheal rings. Portex also market a series of straight white dilators (but not to date in the UK).

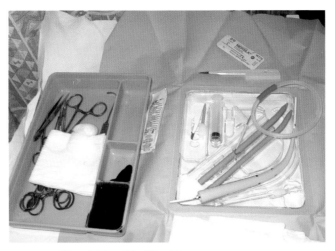

Fig. 7.3 **Blue Rhino kit (Cook).**

There are design differences between these kits in terms of curved or straight dilators, the materials they are made of, and whether multiple serial dilators are used or a single-step dilator as in the Cook's Blue Rhino kit (Figure 7.3). With the sequential dilator kits, the stoma is successively dilated, starting with a 12-French dilator and ending up with a 36-French dilator. The tracheostomy tube itself is introduced into the trachea over an appropriately sized dilator. A recurrent problem with dilation techniques is the step between the introducing dilator and the tracheostomy tube mounted on it. Bevel-tipped tracheostomy tubes have been developed but all tubes end up with a significant step between tube and dilator, in particular with rigid as opposed to flexible tubes. This gives rise to significant resistance during insertion and risk that there is damage to the trachea, in particular disruption of the tracheal rings.

The Blue Rhino is a single-step dilator made by Cook. Portex market a very similar white single-step dilator. There are several advantages over the traditional Ciaglia sequential dilator technique:

1.   The process of dilating up the space between the tracheal rings requires less force. The dilator is hydrophilic and when immersed in water or saline becomes very smooth and allows easy passage of the dilator through tissues. This reduces the likelihood of bleeding and tissue damage.

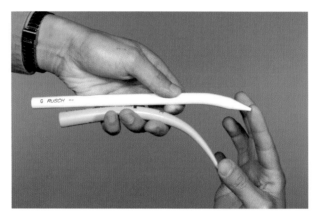

Fig. 7.4 Blue Rhino dilator more flexible than the stiffer Rüsch dilator (white).

2. A single dilatation avoids the spraying of blood in between dilatations. The continuous tamponade reduces bleeding.
3. The increased speed of the technique reduces the time during which the dilators and bronchoscope are obstructing the airway. This reduces the risk of hypercarbia and hypoxia.
4. Traditional dilators are quite stiff and there is a risk of damaging the posterior tracheal wall. The Blue Rhino is flexible and more likely to bend at the appropriate angle to follow the direction of the wire down the trachea (Figure 7.4).

Forceps-based techniques

In 1989, Schachner[4] described a forceps-based technique (Rapitrach). A needle was passed into the trachea and a short guidewire inserted. The forceps (Figure 7.5), which had relatively sharp tips, were passed over the guidewire into the trachea and then opened. The guidewire was removed and the tracheostomy tube and obturator were inserted between the jaws of the forceps. The device was originally designed for emergency use and gave rapid access to the trachea, but the sharp beveled tip was associated with rupture of the tracheostomy tube cuff and there have been reports of the posterior tracheal wall being split. The forceps were often opened inadvertently in pretracheal tissues.

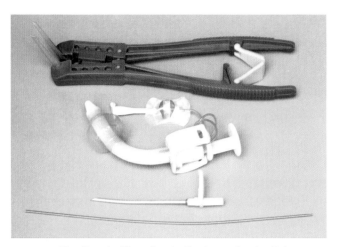

Fig. 7.5 Rapitrach (Surgitech, Sydney, Australia).

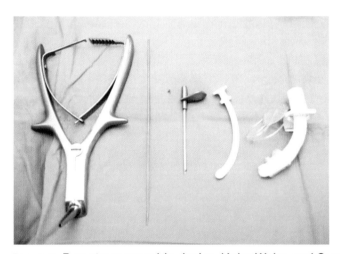

Fig. 7.6 Percutrac: reusable device (John Weiss and Son Ltd, Milton Keynes, UK).

The forceps were available initially as a single use disposable item but subsequently adapted as a reusable kit.[5] Like the Rapitrach, the Percutrac (Figure 7.6) allows rapid access to the trachea over a guidewire. The longer jaws makes pretracheal placement less likely. The kit achieved some success but a number of cases of posterior tracheal and oesophageal damage occurred as a result of the sharp tips of the device, when the operator lost control of the device within the trachea. Once the forceps are opened they can fall away from the guidewire and control is lost. In addition, the tube is not passed over the guidewire. Such devices do not adhere to the concept of the Seldinger technique, when the guidewire stays in place until the successful completion of the procedure. To the authors' knowledge, both the Rapitrach and Percutrac have been withdrawn from the market.

In 1990, Griggs[6] described an alternative technique using dilating forceps, which comprise a pair of Howard-Kelly forceps that have been modified by increasing the curvature and by drilling a central hole from the tip that allows passage of a flexible guidewire (Figure 7.7). The Griggs technique (Portex) is definitely faster, but the Ciaglia serial dilation technique (Cook) is preferred by most operators because it produces gradual, progressive dilation of the stoma with a tamponade effect on stoma vessels and minimal bleeding. It is recommended in the instructions that the forceps are opened both outside the trachea and in the trachea. Verification that the tips of the forceps are within the trachea can be made by pulling them anteriorly. If in the tissues, the skin and subcutaneous tissues will 'tent' outwards. If in the trachea, there will be a firm feeling on trying to pull them outwards. Alternatively, bronchoscopic verification can be used.

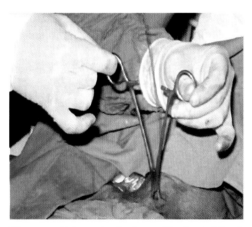

Fig. 7.7 Griggs technique (Portex). The handles of the forceps have been lifted so that the tips of the forceps lie parallel to the long axis of the trachea. The tracheal stoma is being dilated as the handles are separated.

Concerns have been raised with this and other forceps devices including:

1. The risk of over-stretching of the trachea if the forceps handles are opened too widely.
2. The jaws of forceps do not open in a parallel movement.
3. There is no calibration device to tell you how wide the forceps are open.
4. The risk of damage to the posterior tracheal wall.

Forceps techniques may be more advantageous if the patient is awake, as the dilatation procedure may be more comfortable for the patient compared with pushing plastic dilatators inwards.

Fantoni kit

In 1997, Fantoni introduced a translaryngeal approach (Figure 7.8). The translaryngeal technique has a number of theoretical advantages over other techniques because the tracheostomy tube is pulled from inside the trachea to the outside and no external pressure is applied into the trachea from the outside. In addition, as the dilator is an integral part of the tracheostomy tube, there is no step between the two as seen with other kits. There should, therefore, be less potential for damage to the anterior and posterior

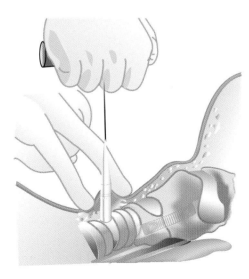

Fig. 7.8 **Fantoni technique (Mallinkrodt). The conal dilator is being pulled out of the trachea.**

tracheal wall. In addition, it can theoretically be used in children and young adults.[7] No other kits currently available are recommended for use in children and the safety of this and other kits in children remains unknown. It is important to realise that even minor degrees of tracheal stenosis in the small paediatric trachea may be significant.

In this technique, the trachea is accessed with a needle under endoscopic control. The original description involved a rigid bronchoscope passed through an unusual rigid straight-cuffed endotracheal tube. The needle is aimed in a cephalad direction and the guidewire passed upwards to appear in either the ET tube, or the patient's mouth. This guidewire is different to traditional guidewires in that it has two different sections bonded together. The first is a traditional soft flexible J-tipped component to pass through the needle up out of the mouth. The second section is made of high tensile steel, which is able to resist considerable traction forces. This strong section is subsequently used to pull the dilator out of the trachea.

The guidewire is pulled out of the mouth and the flexible J-tipped wire component cut off to leave the high tensile wire *in situ*. The latter is passed into the conal dilator and a knot formed, which then attaches the guidewire to the conal dilator. The ET tube is removed and the conal dilator, which has an integral armoured tracheostomy tube attached to it, is pulled down through the larynx and subsequently out of the tracheal wall. Counter-traction can be provided in the neck with pressure from the operator's fingers. Once the conal dilator is pulled out of the neck, it is cut off, leaving the tracheostomy tube *in situ*. However, the tip and cuffed section of this tube faces cephalad and has to be turned round. This is facilitated by the use of a special obturator or the use of a rigid or flexible bronchoscope so that the tip comes to lie facing downwards. A 15 mm connector is attached to the tube and ventilation can then be commenced through the tube and its position confirmed by the usual techniques.

The concept of pulling tubes out of the trachea is attractive conceptually, as it avoids tracheal rings being pushed inwards and enables counter-traction to be applied by the operator's other hand.

However, the whole operative sequence is quite complicated and suffers from a number of disadvantages:

1. The procedure is ideally performed with a rigid bronchoscope. Such bronchoscopes are not widely available in most ICUs. In addition, the bronchoscope has to be passed through a specially designed rigid ET tube, which would be unfamiliar to most intensive care staff and may be difficult or traumatic to insert if laryngoscopy is difficult.
2. The airway is potentially lost on more than one occasion during the tracheostomy procedure. The ET tube needs to be removed in order to allow the conal dilator device to pass down through the larynx and out of the trachea. In addition, the manoeuvres required to turn around the tracheostomy tube from cephalad to caudal direction are not straightforward. The manufacturer of the kit provides a long small-bore (ID 4 mm) ET tube, similar to a microlaryngoscopy tube. This tube can be left *in situ* throughout the procedure to provide some oxygenation and ventilation. All dilation and positioning procedures are performed alongside it. Nevertheless the loss of the airway can be hazardous.
3. The complexity of the kits and associated devices make them expensive compared to other devices.
4. The resultant armoured, adjustable flange, tracheostomy tube is of a rather unusual design with a non-profile cuff very close to its tip. The material of this tube has high coefficient of friction which makes suction catheters difficult to pass.

For all these reasons, despite its theoretical attractions, this kit has not achieved widespread use (Table 7.1).

PercuTwist

The newest dilating device is the screw in PercuTwist® device marketed by Rüsch (Figure 7.9). This kit utilises a self-tapping screw dilator, with the idea that this provides more precise control of dilation, avoiding inward forces that may cause damage to the trachea or other structures. The trachea is accessed with a needle and guidewire as with other techniques. The screw in dilator is

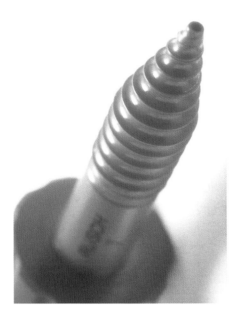

Fig. 7.9 PercuTwist (Rüsch).

screwed into the trachea under bronchoscopic guidance to ensure that the posterior wall of the trachea is not traumatised by screwing the device in too far. Once the tracheal dilation has been performed, the tracheostomy tube is inserted over the guidewire in a similar manner to that employed by other kits.

Experience to date has been limited with this technique. The concept is attractive, but there have already been reports of posterior wall damage from the device.[8] The length of the threaded tapered section is about the diameter of the average adult trachea.

Cricothyroidotomy kits

The cricothyroid membrane has been utilised as a site of access for both small- and larger-bore tracheostomy tubes. Historically, there have been a large series of patients reported in whom the cricothyroid membrane was utilised for long-term tracheostomy as opposed to incisions lower in the trachea. This route was used to avoid contamination of sternotomy wounds following cardiac surgery.[9] In addition, a number of smaller-bore tubes have been

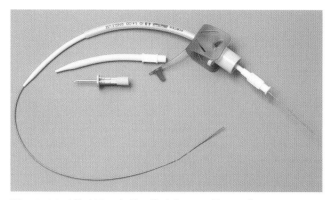

Fig. 7.10 Mini-Trach II – Seldinger (Portex).

developed, both for the treatment of respiratory failure and sputum retention (so-called minitracheostomy kits), and for emergency use. The former is generally in the form of a 4 mm ID non-cuffed tube. These were developed with the idea of enhancing cough and sputum clearance in patients with respiratory failure after surgical procedures. Before the advent of percutaneous tracheostomy, such devices were used regularly in the hope that tracheal intubation or re-intubation in susceptible patients could be avoided. Such procedures were generally performed in awake patients under local anaesthesia.

Initial devices had the minitracheostomy tube mounted on a blunt plastic introducing obturator. It was often difficult to find the trachea following the skin incision due to mobility of the tissues in the neck. Subsequently, the design was improved by utilisation of a Seldinger technique which made it much more reliable (Figure 7.10). Such devices were widely used in the 1970s and 1980s.[10] Their use has declined considerably since the advent of percutaneous tracheostomy techniques that allow the introduction of 8 or 9 mm ID cuffed tracheostomy tubes. Limitations of the minitracheostomy kit (ID 4 mm) include small-bore suction (10 FG), inability to provide CPAP and positive pressure ventilation. There is no cuff to provide airway protection. Their use should only be considered if it is felt that the patient is likely to rapidly improve.

Larger cricothyroidotomy kits (Figure 7.11) have been developed for emergency use (e.g. the Melker device). This is available in the non-cuffed version with a 3.5–6 mm ID tube.

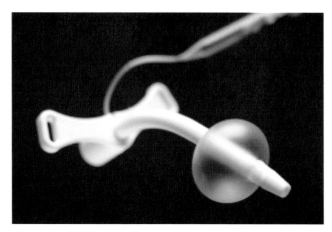

Fig. 7.11 Melker kit (Cook).

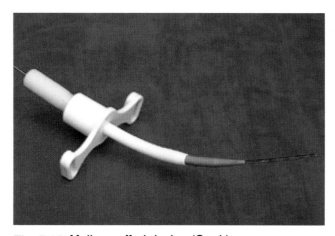

Fig. 7.12 Melker cuffed device (Cook).

More recently, a cuffed version (ID 5 mm) is also available (Figure 7.12). Such devices are widely available in the accident and emergency setting, and also on difficult intubation trolleys in anaesthesia and intensive care units.

References

1 Cook TM. Novel airway devices: spoilt for choice? *Anaesthesia* 2003; **58**: 107–10
2 Paw HGW, Turner S. The current state of percutaneous tracheostomy in intensive care: a postal survey. *Clin Intens Care* 2002; **13**: 95–101
3 Seldinger SI. Catheter replacement of the needle in percutaneous arteriography. *Acta Radiol* 1953; **39**: 368–76

4 Schachner A, Ovil Y, Sidi J, Rogev M, Helibronn Y, Levy MJ. Percutaneous tracheostomy – a new method. *Crit Care Med* 1989; **17**: 1052–6

5 Whittet HB, Marks N, Waldmann C, Douglas S. The 'Percutrac': a minimally invasive percutaneous tracheostomy device. *Minimal Invas Ther* 1993; **2**: 319–24

6 Griggs WM, Worthley LI, Gilligan JE, Thomas PD, Myburg JA. A simple percutaneous tracheostomy technique. *Surg Gynecol Obstet* 1990; **170**: 543–5

7 Fantoni A, Ripamonti D. A non-derivative, non-surgical tracheostomy: the translaryngeal method. *Intens Care Med* 1997; **23**: 386–92

8 Mallick A, Sharma A, Elliot S, Bell D, Vucevic M. Preliminary evaluation of PercuTwist tracheostomy in ICU patients. *Br J Intens Care* 2003; **13**: 6–10

9 Brantigan CO, Grow Sr JB. Cricothyroidotomy: elective use in respiratory problems requiring tracheotomy. *J Thorac Cardiovasc Surg* 1976; **71**: 72–81

10 Ryan DW. Minitracheotomy. *Br Med J* 1990; **300**: 958–9

Tracheostomy Tubes

There is a wide range of tubes available commercially. They incorporate a variety of design features (Box 8.1).

Box 8.1 Design features of tracheostomy tubes

1 Rigid *versus* softer thermoplastic tube
2 Profile *versus* non-profile cuff or non-cuffed
3 Inner liner for ease of cleaning
4 Fenestrations for communication
5 Small channels above the cuff
   (a) to remove pooled secretions above the cuff
   (b) as a gas source (attached to high-pressure source to aid speech)
6 Bevelled end for ease of insertion over dilators
7 Flexible anchoring flange
8 Adjustable flange for longer stem tube
9 PVC/Silver/Silastic materials
10 15 mm external connector/non-standard connector
11 Reinforcement spiral/no reinforcement
12 Ease of suctioning down device
13 Angle of stem 90–120°

The history of such devices has moved from rigid silver tubes to include the presence of an inner liner for ease of cleaning, and fenestrations and valves for communication. Tubes were subsequently made with detachable rubber cuffs. Red rubber tubes with built-in inflatable cuffs followed.

The modern generation of tubes are made out of soft or rigid plastic, or a silicone rubber armoured coil. Intuitively, it would seem sensible, wherever possible, to use as soft and flexible a material as possible, to provide maximum patient comfort and minimise any trauma to the trachea and associated structures. Nevertheless, it is common practice to use rigid tubes in the longer term, in the belief that they keep the stoma open better than flexible materials and are easier to change. Interestingly, it has long been recognised that silver tubes may have an antibacterial effect from the silver oxidising. This concept is now being used in intravenous catheters but has not yet been revisited in airway devices.

Many kits (e.g. Rhino + TRACOE, Rüsch + PercuQuick) now have a tracheostomy tube contained within them. This has the advantage that exact-fitting dilators are provided with the tube. Otherwise, the tubes may not snugly fit dilators. In general, softer tubes will fit dilators much more easily than the more rigid tubes to avoid the shelf-like 'steps' that can be seen between tube and dilator (Figure 8.1).

There are arguments for and against siting longer-term fenestrated tubes at the initiation of tracheostomy in the ICU situation compared with subsequently changing towards such tubes prior to discharge to ward-based care. There have been problems with surgical emphysema in the neck tissues in ventilated patients when the fenestrations do not lie completely within the tracheal lumen. Air under positive pressure can track outwards between the tube and inner liner to exit out of the fenestrations into the neck tissues.

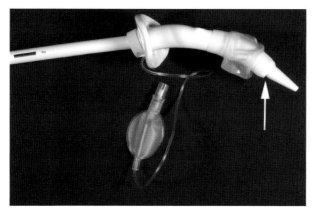

Fig. 8.1 'Step' (white arrow) caused by ill fitting between Shiley tracheostomy tube and Rüsch dilator: the dilator is not the same angle as the rigid tracheostomy tube and is distorting it.

The introduction of high-volume low-pressure profile type cuffs is thought to have reduced the incidence of cuff-related mucosal damage by providing a wider surface area of the trachea for the pressure to be dissipated. Nevertheless, many units do not routinely measure cuff pressures with appropriate devices (Figure 8.2). The cuff pressure should not exceed 25 cm H_2O (18 mmHg) in order to reduce the risk of impaired mucosal perfusion, tissue necrosis and tracheal stenosis. It should also be appreciated that such profile cuffs will not perform optimally if the tracheal tube is too small for an individual patient's trachea. The theoretical attractions of a smaller potentially less traumatic tube, need to be balanced against the inadequate performance of an overstretched profile cuff and too short a stem.

Other cuff designs are available (e.g. foam filled cuffs designed to minimise cuff pressures), but these have not achieved widespread usage to date.

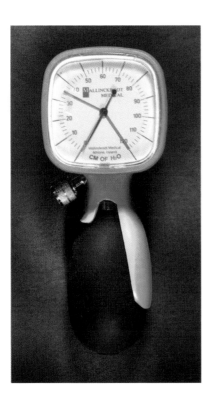

Fig. 8.2 Inflating bulb and pressure gauge used to measure and adjust cuff pressure.

Indications for cuffed tracheostomy tubes, and their disadvantages, are outlined in Boxes 8.2 and 8.3.

- Patient dependent on IPPV or CPAP
- Patients at risk of aspiration

- Excessive cuff pressure may reduce perfusion of the tracheal mucosa leading to tracheal stenosis
- Patient is unable to speak with a non-fenestrated tube
- The act of swallowing may be impaired

Tracheostomy tubes with an inner cannula

Secretions can adhere to the inside of the tracheostomy tube lumen, causing a reduction in the internal diameter and increasing the work of breathing and/or obstructing the patient's airway. To prevent this from occurring, a single lumen tracheostomy tube (without an inner cannula) should be changed every 7–14 days. Such frequent tube changes can cause patient discomfort, trauma and loss of the airway. A tracheostomy tube with an inner cannula can minimise these risks and remain in place for up to 30 days. The inner cannula can be cleaned or changed regularly. These two-piece tracheostomy tubes may be fenestrated or non-fenestrated. The fenestrated tube allows airflow through the vocal cords when the tube is occluded or a speaking valve is attached.

There are several points to bear in mind with these tubes:

- The diameter of the inner lumen will be reduced by at least 1–2 mm. This may increase the patient's effort of breathing and delay weaning.
- Patients who are at risk of aspiration or are on positive pressure ventilation should not have a fenestrated tube unless

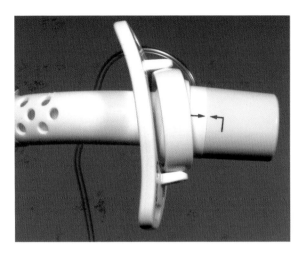

Fig. 8.3 Alignment of a 'twist-lock' tracheostomy tube.

a non-fenestrated inner cannula is used to block off the fenestrations.

- When suctioning a patient with a fenestrated tracheostomy tube, the fenestrated inner cannula should be replaced with the non-fenestrated inner cannula *in situ* to occlude the fenestrations and guide the suction catheter into the trachea.
- The reusable inner cannula requires at least daily cleaning (unless precluded by severe ventilator-dependence) to prevent the build-up of biofilm on the inner surface. When removing the inner cannula for inspection or cleaning, the 15 mm connector should also be removed. If the patient is ventilator dependent, a spare inner cannula must be inserted to allow for connection to the breathing circuit (resuscitation bag or ventilator circuit).
- In tracheostomy tubes using the 'twist-lock' locking system, the lines or dots on the two tubes must be aligned to lock it in (Figure 8.3). Attending staff must be aware of how such devices work. Repeated problems can occur when staff fail to understand how inner and outer tubes fit together and how such tubes require the inner liner *in situ* to attach to a resuscitation bag or ventilator circuit. To prevent the system from accidentally unlocking, it is best to place the ventilator on the patient's left side, thus the weight of the catheter mount with ventilator tubing will tend to twist the inner tube in a clockwise direction, ensuring it remains locked.

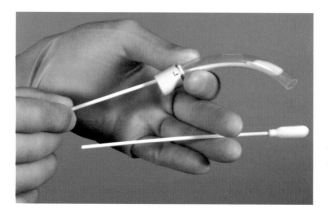

TRACOE® cleaning swab. A long, flexible plastic handle with a soft polyurethane sponge attached to its end.

Cleaning the reusable inner cannula

- Remove the inner cannula and replace it with a temporary inner cannula
- Rinse the inner cannula with sterile 0.9% saline
- To loosen any encrustations, use a TRACOE® cleaning swab (Figure 8.4)

Tracheostomy tubes with disposable inner cannula are an alternative. The advantages of using disposable inner cannula includes:

- Cost-effective (avoids cleaning solution, cotton buds, gloves, etc.), but the tubes are not as cheap as might be anticipated.
- Nursing time.
- Infection control risks.

The disadvantages of tracheostomy tubes with disposable inner cannula are:

- High cost.
- Small size and unobtrusive design means that inexperienced staff may not recognise the inner liner is *in situ*: some only have small ring pull to indicate the inner tube is *in situ*.

Tracheostomy tube with an adjustable flange

Tracheostomy tubes with an adjustable flange are specifically designed for patients whose trachea is deeper than usual below the skin and other tissues in the neck. These may include those who have distorted anatomy within the neck and the obese patient. The adjustable flange means that the stem can be adjusted to the desired length and the intratracheal section of tube and cuff lies in a comfortable parallel position within the trachea (see Chapter 11: Complications).

The choice of tracheostomy tube

There is a dearth of evidence for the recommendation of one tube over another. Certain caveats apply, however:

1. In general, flexible tubes are easier to insert over percutaneous dilators than rigid tubes.
2. Patients with a thick or fat neck, goitres or other anatomical abnormalities are likely to need a long stem or adjustable flange tracheostomy tube. Standard length tubes have a rather short stem.
3. The longer-term patient, particularly when breathing spontaneously, is likely to benefit from a removable inner liner and speaking fenestrations.
4. If anatomy is significantly distorted, flexible armoured tubes may be helpful.

Clinicians should have a low threshold to change tubes. The device first chosen may subsequently prove unsatisfactory and may benefit from being changed. If there are concerns regarding its position, then fibreoptic endoscopy through the tube and from above via the larynx will ensure optimal configuration.

There are companies that custom-make tubes at relatively short notice for the patient with anatomical abnormalities. In addition, there are specialist products like double lumen endobronchial devices for right or left placement (Rüsch). These are, in essence, shorter versions of translaryngeal double lumen endobronchial tubes.

Speaking aids for tracheostomy

There are a number of speaking aids to improve verbal communication for the patient with a tracheostomy. Deflation of the cuff may allow enough air to pass through he cords to allow speech. If the patient is still ventilated, speech can be facilitated by allowing expired air past the deflated cuff. Some patients will strain to build up pressure to cause a leak and allow speech. Alternatively, manually obstructing airflow out from the exhalational limb of a CPAP or ventilator circuit will achieve a similar effect.

The presence of fenestrations allows the air to pass up through the larynx, even when the cuff of the tube is inflated. An alternative is to use tubes where air or oxygen can be provided by a separate channel from a pressurised source to allow communication, even if the ventilator circuit is unbreached. The latter usually only allows the patient to whisper and requires practice to develop.

There are a number of other valvular mechanisms that fit on to the external portion of the tracheostomy tube to prevent exhalation back out of the tracheostomy tube and up through the larynx. Such devices are generally used in the longer-term patient rather than the sicker ICU patient. There are practical difficulties in dealing with alarm functions on ICU ventilators if such devices are used.

Other vibrational aids (e.g. a tone generator in laryngectomy patients) may also be used. These need practice and are really only useful for the longer-term patient. Other obvious techniques include lip reading, text boards, and electronic writing aids.

Further reading

Manzano JL, *et al.* Verbal communication of ventilator dependent patients. *Crit Care Med* 1993; **21**: 512–7

Leder SB. Importance of verbal communication for the ventilator dependent patient. *Chest* 1990; **98**: 792–3

Wilson DJ. Tracheal Appliances. In Grillo HC (Ed) *Surgery of the Trachea and Bronchi.* 2004: BC Decker Inc; Hamilton, Ontario, pp 735–48

9 Anaesthesia and Surgical Techniques

General considerations

Two trained operators are required: one with adequate training in percutaneous tracheostomy and management of complications (see below) and the other skilled in anaesthesia and other aspects of airway care. Procedures should ideally be performed during normal working hours to ensure backup from senior staff and other specialists should any complications occur.

Consent/assent is generally sought from the patient or relatives. Most patients requiring intensive care support will not be deemed capable of giving consent, but may be able to understand a verbal/written explanation of what is to happen next. The position of third party consent in this context is legally debatable at the current time in the UK. As the majority of procedures are electively performed, to aid weaning, it is sensible to let family members know that the procedure is to be performed. Families are often very distressed if procedures performed without their knowledge subsequently develop complications. The need for such discussions provides an ideal opportunity to assess and discuss overall chances of survival, plans for weaning and further care. Reasonable figures for quoted mortality or serious morbidity would be 1–2% and 10–15%, respectively. Such risks need to be balanced against the risks of further prolonged translaryngeal intubation and the side effects of continued administration of sedative and analgesic drugs.

Some practical aspects of care should be considered when planning a percutaneous tracheostomy procedure (Box 9.1).

> Box 9.1 **Checklist of some practical considerations**
>
> - Ensure patients, their families and other attending staffs are aware of the procedure
> - Stop NG feeding 4–6 h before the procedure and aspirate NG tube immediately prior to procedure
> - Ensure heparin prophylaxis has been given >12 h previously (the evening before, e.g. 18:00 h if morning procedure planned)
> - Stop continuous haemofiltration 4 h before the procedure
> - Check platelets and clotting (correct or delay if INR >1.5 or platelets <80)
> - Assess potential problems for anaesthesia and surgery (see below)
> - Place a rolled up towel or sandbag between shoulder blades or extend head and neck over existing pillow

Anaesthetic considerations

The translaryngeal airway

An anaesthetist or other suitably trained operator is required to ensure that the translaryngeal airway is not lost, and that the patient is adequately oxygenated, ventilated and anaesthetised for the duration of the procedure. There is a risk that the interest generated in performing the procedure of percutaneous tracheostomy may divert attention from the equally important aspects of anaesthesia and airway care. Anaesthetists/intensivists should not leave junior inexperienced trainees unattended to manage the translaryngeal airway and anaesthesia. Dislodgement of the translaryngeal tube is common, as the tube has to be pulled back into the laryngeal inlet to provide access to the trachea with introducing needles and dilators. If the patient is difficult to intubate due to glottic oedema or pre-existing abnormalities, translaryngeal re-intubation may prove impossible. Check the upper airway for potential difficulty in re-intubation using direct laryngoscopy, leaving the ET tube *in situ*. If you anticipate difficulty and this is not your area of expertise, call for senior help. There have been a number of hypoxic incidents recorded in such situations. The airway can be protected by the passage of a gum elastic bougie or airway exchange catheter through the ET tube via a bronchoscopic connector (Figure 9.1). This allows for continued ventilation through the ET tube alongside

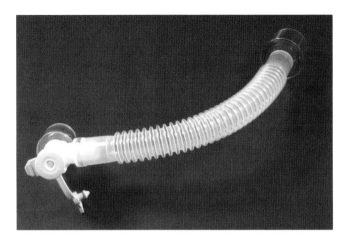

Fig. 9.1 Catheter mount with 15 mm connector with access port.

the bougie. The ET tube can be moved backwards and forwards out of the way of the operator, and the bougie left within the trachea until the tracheostomy tube is definitively in place. Alternatively, a fibreoptic bronchoscope down the tube will perform a similar (albeit very expensive if damaged) function.

Other airway devices have been used for this indication. The laryngeal mask airway (LMA) has an established role, and may be the technique of choice, provided that the patient does not require high-inflation pressures or have a significant risk of pulmonary aspiration.[1] The use of the LMA or the Pro-Seal LMA[2] allows all airway devices, including fibreoptic scopes, to be kept out of the surgical area of the trachea. Its large bore allows easy ventilation with a bronchoscope *in situ*. As it sits above the larynx, better views of the glottis (to assess larynx and cord damage), cricoid and first ring are obtained compared with those seen through a translaryngeal tube. Oesophageal obturator devices such as the Combitube (Figure 9.2) have also been used, but cause considerable distortion of structures around the airway and we would not recommend routine use for this procedure.[3]

One of the authors (Andrew R. Bodenham) knows of a case of awareness where inadequate anaesthetic had been administered to a patient with a high spinal cord injury who was fully conscious and in pain whilst undergoing percutaneous tracheostomy. It is likely that other cases of awareness have gone unreported. Patients *must* be given adequate amounts of intravenous or volatile anaesthetic

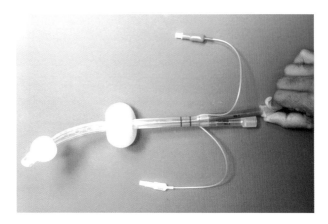

Fig. 9.2 Combitube.

agents, in addition to a suitable muscle relaxant. Generous administration of local anaesthetic containing adrenaline will provide local anaesthesia, post-operative pain relief and help haemostasis. It is not sufficient to give boluses of propofol and a muscle relaxant alone. To date, the authors are not aware of any medicolegal cases involving awareness in the ICU situation. It is accepted that it is impractical and unsafe to render patients unconscious throughout their stay on ICU. Nevertheless awareness, in the context of a planned, painful surgical procedure such as percutaneous tracheostomy, is unacceptable and would not be defensible in court. The same care and attention is required as for standard anaesthetic practice in theatre (Table 9.1).

Anaesthetic sequence

One suggested anaesthetic technique is as follows:

- Induce anaesthesia with fentanyl and propofol.
- Paralyse the patient with atracurium and maintain on a propofol infusion.
- Volume-cycled ventilation with a PEEP of 5 cm H_2O and 100% oxygen can be adjusted to give the desired $ETCO_2$.
- Extend the head by pushing the pillow under the shoulders.
- Check the airway using direct laryngoscopy, suck out secretions, and assess any potential difficulty of re-intubation.

Table 9.1 **Suggested anaesthetic checklist**

Equipment	Have standard intubation equipment ready and checked
	Oropharyngeal airways
	Two working laryngoscopes
	Suction with Yankauer and large-bore suction catheters (12–16 FG)
	Selection of ET tubes of different sizes (7–9 ID)
	Bougies/airway exchange catheter
	LMA sizes 3, 4 and 5
	Magill forceps
	Sterilised fibreoptic bronchoscope, suction and light source
	Self-inflating bag and mask
	Resuscitation equipment and drugs
Drugs	Fentanyl 100–200 µg
	Propofol infusion
	Atracurium
	Lidocaine 2% with 1 in 200,000 epinephrine
Ventilation	Consider volume-cycled ventilation
	↑ FiO_2 to 100%
	PEEP of 5 cm H_2O
Monitoring	BP
	SpO_2
	ECG
	Tidal volume
	Peak inspiratory pressure
	PEEP
	Capnography ($ETCO_2$)

- Pull back the ET tube under direct vision: once the cuff of the ET tube has been withdrawn sufficiently, the tip of the bronchoscope should be positioned so that it is protected within the ET tube (beware damage of bronchoscope through Murphy's eye (Figure 9.3).

Where appropriate, the ET tube may be replaced by an LMA. The translaryngeal airway must be maintained until correct tracheostomy tube placement in the trachea has been confirmed (see below). Rapid re-intubation by the translaryngeal route *must* be achievable as this is the standard rescue option if the tracheostomy procedure proves difficult in any way.

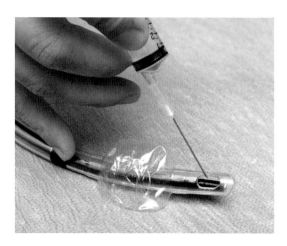

Fig. 9.3 Potential needle damage to bronchoscope via Murphy's eye.

Surgical techniques

Inspection of the neck may reveal venous or arterial pulsations, a prominent thyroid gland and/or old surgical scars. Assess the overall size of the patient and how thick their neck is; are they likely to need a larger-bore or long-stemmed tube? Palpation may reveal arterial pulsations, either in the neck or transmitted from the great vessels in the thoracic inlet. The outline of the trachea, and thyroid and cricoid cartilages can usually be felt. Plain chest X-rays may reveal tracheal narrowing or deviation, intrathoracic goitres or other abnormalities. Further information may be available from other incidental imaging (e.g. CT or MRI of the cervical spine or chest). Ultrasound can give further information on soft tissues, in particular blood vessels and thyroid gland.

Inexperienced operators should *not* be left alone to perform the procedure. An experienced operator, scrubbed up and present at the bedside, should supervise initial procedures.

Practicalities
Operators should ensure that they have the following items ready:

- Sterile gown, gloves and surgical drapes.
- Mask eye protection (to protect from aerosolisation of blood and secretions).

- Antiseptic cleansing solution.
- Local anaesthetic and sterile 0.9% saline.
- Tracheostomy tubes, range of diameters and lengths.
- Percutaneous tracheostomy kit plus another spare kit.
- Syringes and needles.
- Sterile forceps (Spencer Wells or curved mosquito).
- Basic surgical instrumentation (e.g. cut down set).
- Anchoring suture (e.g. long curved 2-0 silk).
- Tape to tie tube *in situ*.
- Absorbable suture for haemostasis (e.g. 3-0 vicryl).
- Sterile lubricant.
- Suction catheters to pass down tracheostomy tube.
- A sterile pot for sterile saline (to clean bronchoscope).

Surgical incision

The skin incision should be just skin-deep. Any deeper, and there is a risk of cutting into vessels (e.g. anterior jugular veins). A head-up tilt of up to 30° will reduce distension of neck veins. The preferred insertion sites are between either the first and second or the second and third tracheal rings. There is a higher incidence of tracheal stenosis if the insertion site is higher, i.e. between the cricoid and first tracheal ring. Below the third ring, there is a higher risk of bleeding from puncturing great vessels, the highly vascular thyroid isthmus and occasionally, the pyramidal lobe. In practice, many patients requiring tracheostomy on ICU will have a short neck and hyperinflated chest from COPD. Such patients have very limited space in their neck. The incision will have to be made immediately above the sternal notch and the tracheal stoma sited between the first and second rings. A horizontal 1–1.5 cm incision is adequate. (see Chapter 13: Tips and Tricks).

Blunt dissection

The value of initial dissection prior to needle and guidewire placement has been debated. Arguments *for* this procedure include:

- If blood vessels are damaged, it is preferable that this occurs prior to the trachea being opened, thereby stopping the risk of blood draining into the trachea.

It also offers the opportunity for the operator to insert the index or another finger into the tissues to assess:

- The presence of arterial pulsations should alert the operator, unless transmitted from normally placed great vessels in upper chest.
- The lie of the trachea – is it in the midline? Does it descend steeply backwards into the chest?
- The level of thyroid, cricoid cartilages and lower tracheal rings.

Early dissection also reduces the forces required for subsequent passage of dilators.

The authors recommend the use of a pair of curved forceps (e.g. Spencer Wells or mosquito forceps) for blunt dissection of the superficial muscle layers in a transverse plane. Vertical dilatation using the forceps will risk tearing the vessels. It is important not to dilate the trachea itself using the forceps because of the risk of tearing it. Other operators omit such steps and only incise the skin immediately prior to dilation of the tissues.

Needle entry

Needle placement can be guided by digital palpation of the trachea or transillumination of the tissues from the light of a bronchoscope (Figure 9.4). Needle entry into the tracheal lumen is confirmed by aspiration of air (Figure 9.5c) and can be verified using a bronchoscope or capnography. Alternatively, respiratory mucus may be aspirated. If air is aspirated, the operator should not automatically assume that the needle is correctly placed in the trachea because it could be in the lung, or the cuff of the ET tube. If it is suspected that the ET tube has been hit, the operator should ask the anaesthetist to

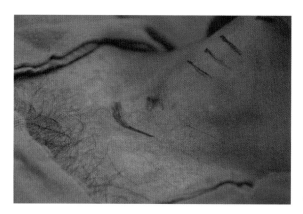

Fig. 9.4 Transillumination to guide needle placement.

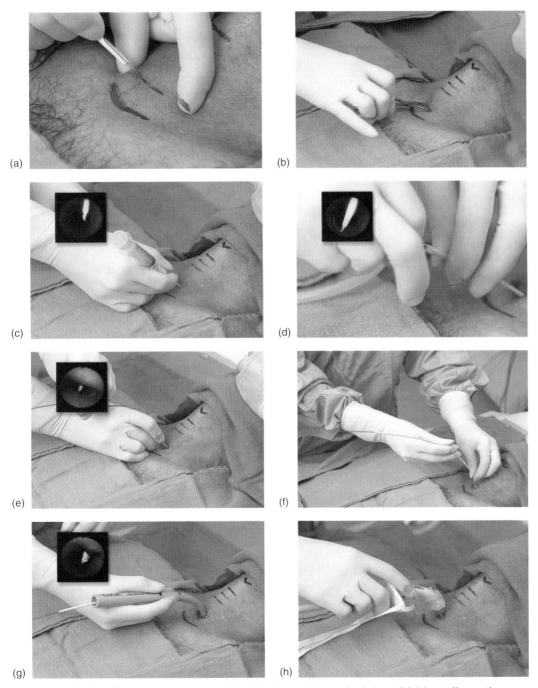

Fig. 9.5 Steps in the dilatation sequence: (a) skin deep 1.5 cm incision; (b) blunt dissection with curved forceps; (c) needle entry into trachea; (d) insertion of guidewire; (e) initial dilator; (f) insertion of guiding catheter over guidewire; (g) dilatation with Blue Rhino dilator; (h) insertion of tracheostomy tube with loading dilator. Thumbnail images show bronchoscopic views.

gently move the ET tube – they will then be able to feel and see the needle move. The operator should ensure that the puncture is in the midline and between the tracheal rings. Damage to the tracheal rings or cricoid may result in a higher incidence of tracheal stenosis. If difficulties are encountered in finding the tracheal lumen or achieving a midline needle placement, the operator should consider using a green needle as a seeker needle in a similar fashion to vascular access procedures. The sharp, narrow-diameter needle causes minimal bleeding and enters the trachea easily. Once correctly sited, it can be used as a guide for the larger introducing needle and cannula.

Debate exists about the relative merits of using needle alone or needle plus cannula. Many kits offer the option of using either. The cannula is prone to kinking and may need to be carefully withdrawn to allow the guidewire to pass. Bronchoscopy is increasingly used to visualise the needle puncture and subsequent dilatation. This can reduce the risk of damage to the trachea, particularly to the posterior tracheal wall.

It is possible for guidewires to be misplaced by passing upwards within the trachea or downwards underneath the tracheal mucosa. Some kits have a plastic stiffener/thickener device to enhance the guiding effect of the guidewire.

Dilation sequence

The operator should ensure that the guidewire is correctly sited and passing towards the carina. The patient will often cough as the guidewire touches the carina if the patient is incompletely paralysed. Dilation is started in most kits with a small short dilator passed over the guidewire (Figure 9.5e). There is a characteristic give on the entry of the shoulder of each dilator as it is passed into the trachea. If resistance is felt, the dilator should be withdrawn and the process reconsidered. Dilators should not be passed further inwards, or deeper, once resistance decreases. Any further insertion is pointless and may risk trauma to the posterior tracheal wall. Experienced operators understand the direction that dilators must take. The tip has to pass directly backwards to enter the trachea and then be redirected downwards to follow the course of the trachea. If problems with air leaks or heavy bleeding occur, the operator should consider leaving the appropriate dilator *in situ* to seal the hole.

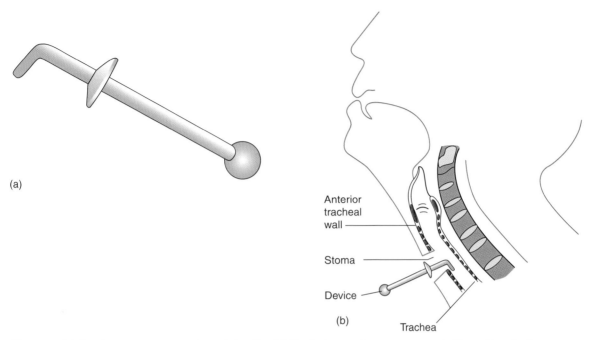

Fig. 9.6 (a) Device to measure stomal depth. (b) Technique of measurement. Place the device through the stoma and hook it onto the anterior tracheal wall; then mark at the skin to determine the depth of the stoma track. Modified with permission from Grillo HC (Ed). *Surgery of the Trachea and Bronchi*. 2004: BC Decker Inc; Hamilton, Ontario.

Passage of the tracheostomy tube

The appropriate sized dilator/obturator and tracheostomy tube should be chosen to minimise the 'step' between dilator and tube. There will be further resistance to passage of the dilator when the tracheostomy tube is mounted on it and a slight twisting motion may aid passage through the tissues. If the tube feels too tight, the operator should consider passing a larger dilator or converting to a smaller-bore tracheostomy tube.

Excessive force must not be used. The operator should be prepared to abandon the occasional procedure rather than risk major tracheal damage. Secure the airway with translaryngeal intubation and re-assess the situation with endoscopy and consider ENT referral. Occasional patients will develop a flap of tissue that may require surgical assistance for tube placement.

Note the depth from skin to trachea. This can be measured (Figure 9.6) The stem of a standard 8–9 mm ID tracheostomy tube is approximately 2–3 cm in length. If the trachea is deeper than this, a long-stemmed adjustable flange tube will be required in order for the tube to lie comfortably and safely within the neck tissues and trachea.

Verification of tube placement in the trachea

There are a number of ways to verify correct tube placement within the trachea (Box 9.2). It is not only a question of ability to oxygenate and ventilate the patient but also of achieving the optimal tube placement to ensure patient comfort and limit any tube-related damage to the trachea. The limitations of each verification technique should be appreciated. Patients who are ventilated on 100% oxygen and have good lung function may take several minutes to desaturate following tracheal tube misplacement. Chest auscultation/movements have been repeatedly discredited as a sign of correct tube placement in the context of translaryngeal intubation in other anaesthetic scenarios. Suction catheters can obviously pass down false passages.

Box 9.2 Verification of tube placement in the trachea

Reliable
- $ETCO_2$ trace
- Bronchoscopy through tube
- Bronchoscopy above tube
- Sustained maintenance of SaO_2

Less reliable
- Chest movements/auscultation
- Passage of suction catheters
- Chest X-ray (AP/lateral)
- Tidal volume
- Airway pressure

Tube position should be verified with bronchoscopy above the tracheostomy tube and through it. Visualisation from above will confirm that the tube is in trachea and that there is an adequate length of tube to allow the cuff to sit in a comfortable position in parallel with the tracheal wall. If the tube looks too short, it should be replaced with a longer-stem, adjustable flange tube. Tracheal damage e.g. fracture rings/tears that might later require follow-up or surgical attention. Any damage to the larynx from translaryngeal intubation should also be looked for carefully. Bronchoscopy through the tube can be used to verify that there is no kinking and that the correct intratracheal position has been achieved, with the end hole parallel to the trachea. Checks should be made to ensure that the tracheostomy tube is not too low and has adequate clearance of the carina. The presence of any blood or secretions, which could subsequently block the airway, should also be looked for and removed.

Chest X-ray

A chest X-ray is routinely requested post-insertion of the tracheostomy tube for several reasons (Box 9.3). A chest X-ray can only show the tracheostomy tube in a relative projection to the gas shadow of the trachea. Paratracheal placement may not be evident if the tube is only partially inserted, or is anterior to the trachea on anteroposterior (AP) chest X-ray, or lateral to the trachea on lateral X-ray. The chest X-ray also ensures the correct position of the nasogastric (NG) tube before feeding is commenced. The place of routine chest X-ray after uncomplicated open tracheostomy has been studied and suggested to be unnecessary unless indicated by physiological deterioration or other clinical signs.[4] It is likely that similar considerations apply to uncomplicated percutaneous techniques.[5]

Box 9.3 Reasons for requesting chest X-ray after insertion of tracheostomy

- To exclude pneumothorax and surgical emphysema
- To check the correct position of the tracheostomy tube
- To check the correct position of the NG tube

Securing the tracheostomy tube

Tapes should be attached to secure the tube when the neck is restored to a neutral position. Some clinicians also place retaining sutures for extra security. One disadvantage of sutures is that dressing changes may be more difficult. There are a number of commercially available devices to assist in securing tubes and allowing easy changes of dressings (Figure 9.7).

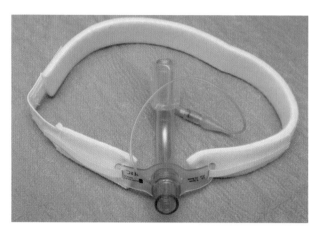

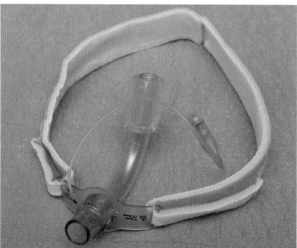

Fig. 9.7 Ties available to secure the tracheostomy tube.

Training and accreditation

The introduction of percutaneous tracheostomy has been somewhat haphazard, in common with other new medical technologies. Initially, there were suggestions that these procedures should only be performed by ENT surgeons or other surgeons capable of repairing any inadvertent damage to the trachea or major blood vessels. This would only be true if very senior ENT, cardiothoracic or head and neck surgeons were to perform the procedures. The surgical trainee is not competent to perform sternotomy or other salvage procedures in the case of major, life-threatening haemorrhage. This argument is therefore somewhat illogical – similar arguments could be put forward for management of the upper airway. The reality is that percutaneous techniques can be safely performed by anaesthetists or intensive care physicians providing they have had adequate training.

There are issues of competence for both the percutaneous tracheostomy procedure and management of complications. The authors would suggest that basic competence in one technique would be achieved in 10–20 procedures if the operator has had no previous experience. Experience with one kit or open surgical technique is likely to accelerate the learning curves for other percutaneous tracheostomy kits. Training needs to encompass the indications and practicalities of undertaking the procedure. In addition, all operators need competence in airway management, chest X-ray interpretation, bronchoscopy, chest drain placement, suturing and haemostasis.

Initially, procedures should be restricted to those with normal anatomy, coagulation and respiratory function until competence is achieved. Procedures should be performed on the ICU, in the anaesthetic room of theatres or in the theatres themselves, depending on the local situation. The authors would not normally undertake such procedures on a general ward. It is debatable whether practitioners need separate training and accreditation for each individual kit. Most institutions will try to restrict the variety of different kits held in stock, so that their staff can become familiar with using one particular kit. There is also some debate as to how widely such procedures should be taught. Clearly, most doctors working longer term on ICU would benefit from being able to do these procedures. Whether every anaesthetic trainee, for instance, needs such skills remains a matter of debate. The authors feel that it is important for all junior anaesthetists to be able to access the trachea with guidewires. Such skills may be life-saving when presented with the *'can't intubate, can't ventilate'* scenario. If practitioners have previous experience of percutaneous tracheostomy, they may well feel able to step in and make a significant clinical impact by performing a percutaneous tracheostomy or some other invasive airway procedure. It is vital that these skills are taught in an elective scenario first.

The popularity of percutaneous tracheostomy has resulted in an increased proportion of ICU patients undergoing tracheostomy earlier.[6] This has also resulted in a decline in open surgical tracheostomy, with an obvious impact on the training opportunities for surgeons.

Documentation

All procedures should be documented in the notes. In the unit of one of the authors (Henry G.W. Paw), a folder is kept aside to record every tracheostomy (both percutaneous and open surgical) to allow for a continuous audit and follow-up (see Appendices 1 and 2).

References

1 Dosemeci L, Yilmaz M, Gürpinar F, Ramazanoglu A. The use of the laryngeal mask airway as an alternative to the endotracheal tube during percutaneous dilatational tracheostomy. *Intens Care Med* 2002; **28**: 63–7

2 Craven RM, Laver SR, Cook TM, Nolan JP. Use of the Pro-Seal LMA facilitates percutaneous dilatational tracheostomy. *Can J Anaesth* 2003; **50**: 718–20

3 Mallick A, Quinn AC, Bodenham AR, Vucevic M. Use of the Combitube for airway maintenance during percutaneous dilatational tracheostomy. *Anaesthesia* 1998; **53**: 249–55

4 Tyroch AH. Routine chest radiograph is not indicated after open tracheostomy. *Am Surg* 2002; **68**: 80–2

5 Datta D. The utility of chest radiographs following percutaneous tracheostomy. *Chest* 2003; **123**: 1603–6

6 Simpson TP, Day CJE, Jewkes CF, Manara AR. The impact of percutaneous tracheostomy on intensive care unit practice and training. *Anaesthesia* 1999; **54**: 186–9

Equipment to Aid Percutaneous Tracheostomy

Percutaneous tracheostomy is a relatively simple, quick and cost-effective procedure. Despite its relative simplicity, there are potential risks centred on misplacement of the needle and guidewire, with subsequent damage to paratracheal structures. To minimise these risks, various aids have been introduced over the years. These include bronchoscopy, ultrasound and capnography.

The role of bronchoscopy

The routine use of fibreoptic bronchoscopy guidance has increased from 30% in 1998[1] to 80.6% in 2002.[2] There is little doubt that bronchoscopy has improved the safety of percutaneous tracheostomy, despite the lack of controlled trials. Initially, the flexible fibreoptic bronchoscope can be used to identify the most appropriate level for the tracheostomy via bronchoscopic transillumination of the trachea (Figure 10.1). The scope can then be used to verify accurate placement of the needle in the midline between the desired tracheal rings (Figure 10.2). It can subsequently be used to verify the satisfactory

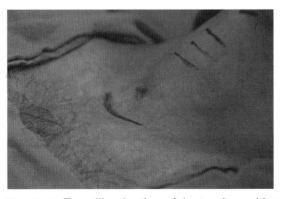

Fig. 10.1 Transillumination of the trachea with a bronchoscope.

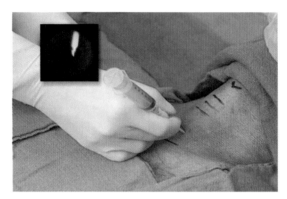

Fig. 10.2 **Needle in the midline between the first and second tracheal rings.**

placement of the guidewire prior to tracheal dilatation and to confirm satisfactory positioning of the tracheostomy tube. Endoscopy also provides a very good teaching aid.

A camera system and large monitor is required so that the operator can see directly what he or she is doing with instrumentation and not rely on the interpretation of another observer. Equally, some competence is required from the person controlling the bronchoscope to achieve adequate visualisation of the upper trachea and operative site without losing the airway. The authors have found that the practice of fibreoptic bronchoscopy in tracheostomy procedures improves trainees' skills in utilising such instrumentation. In particular, if a laryngeal mask is used to secure the airway, one has to negotiate the fibreoptic scope through the glottis and into the trachea. This manoeuvre has obvious similarities to fibreoptic intubation either with or without a laryngeal mask *in situ*.

Accuracy of blind placement

Blind tracheal puncture is inexact. In a cadaveric study,[3] only 45% of the attempts to cannulate the trachea between the first and second tracheal rings were successful, only 15% entered the trachea in the midline and 30% punctured the thyroid isthmus. The authors believe that the use of bronchoscopy may increase the accuracy of needle placement and reduce or avoid many of the complications associated with percutaneous tracheostomy. A study comparing percutaneous tracheostomy performed with and without bronchoscopic guidance[4] found that more serious complications (one tension pneumothorax causing death and two posterior tracheal perforations) occurred when bronchoscopy was not used.

The presence of a fibreoptic bronchoscope within the lumen of the translaryngeal tube seriously reduces the space available for ventilation. This may lead to progressive hypercarbia and hypoxia as a consequence of hypoventilation, which may be particularly troublesome in the more unstable patient or those with already raised intracranial pressure.[5] The role of bronchoscopy in this situation is still debated. Some units use it routinely in all cases, and other units use it more selectively. Hypoventilation can be minimised by using a small diameter bronchoscope, reducing procedure time and using pressure control ventilation.

Bronchoscopy will confirm correct placement of needles, guidewire and dilators in the trachea. It will not always prevent damage to the tracheal wall, however, as damage may only be recognised after it has happened. It cannot visualise the trachea immediately adjacent to the tracheostomy tube and its cuff. In addition, it does not give any information about the presence of blood vessels or other structures outside the trachea.

Care must be taken with introducing needles, as they can very easily produce expensive damage to a fibreoptic bronchoscope. Visualisation is better through a laryngeal mask airway (LMA), which has a larger diameter tube and allows good visualisation of the vocal cords, glottis, and first and second tracheal rings. The scope can be kept further out of the trachea, thus reducing the risk of damage from introducing needles.

Hypoxaemia is the greatest concern in mechanically ventilated patients undergoing fibreoptic bronchoscopy. Some decrease in PaO_2 is inevitable, so most clinicians would avoid performing the procedure in patients requiring an $FiO_2 > 0.6$. Achieving optimal oxygenation during fibreoptic bronchoscopy in the ventilated patient involves several considerations. The effective tidal volume and PEEP must be monitored and maintained as both may be reduced by leaks around the scope. The use of in-circuit bronchoscopic connector allows uninterrupted mechanical ventilation and oxygen delivery during bronchoscopy.

The bronchoscope narrows the lumen of the ET tube (Figure 10.3) and increases both the inspiratory and expiratory resistance. This may lead

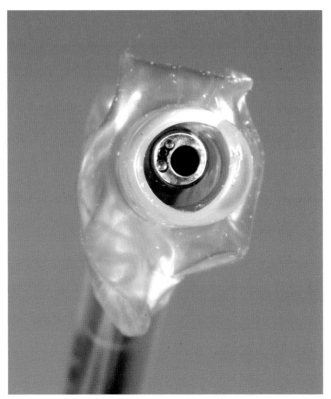

Fig. 10.3 Bronchoscope inside ET tube.

to a pressure-limited decrease in tidal volume because of high-peak inspiratory pressures. For these reasons, many clinicians prefer a volume-cycled mode of ventilation in an attempt to maintain an adequate tidal volume in the presence of higher airways pressures. Auto-PEEP may be generated during fibreoptic bronchoscopy, particularly with smaller ET tubes, when the increased expiratory resistance results in incomplete lung emptying.Other factors may also contribute to the hypoxia, including a reduction in functional residual capacity (FRC) and loss of PEEP during suctioning (which should be intermittent and for short periods only). Passing the scope into bronchi supplying a non-diseased lung may worsen any ventilation–perfusion mismatch already present, as may the instillation of saline for bronchoalveolar lavage. The net effect is to increase the A:a O_2 gradient with the development of hypoxaemia. Hypercarbia is a rare complication of fibreoptic bronchoscopy but the potential for inadequate alveolar ventilation exists, particularly during longer procedures. Hypercapnia can increase ICP in susceptible patients.

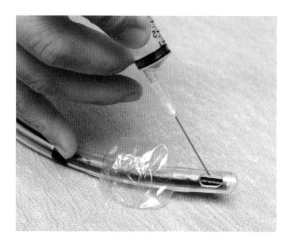

Fig. 10.4 Needle potentially causing damage to bronchoscope through Murphy's eye.

Standard-sized adult scopes may not pass down an ET tube smaller than 8 mm ID. Consider the temporary use of a larger ET tube if appropriate to accommodate the fibrescope. Alternatively, the smaller diameter intubating bronchoscopes used in anaesthetic practice, or paediatric scopes can be used.

A rather expensive complication is damage to the fibreoptic bronchoscope caused by the initial needle insertion. Keeping the bronchoscope within the ET tube provides no guarantee against preventing damage to the bronchoscope, as the needle can sneak in through the Murphy's eye (Figure 10.4), when either the ET tube is too far down the trachea or the site of needle insertion is too high up the neck. An alternative is the use of rigid bronchoscopes which are protected in a metal tube (see Fantoni kit, p. 55). One of the authors (Andrew R. Bodenham) is currently exploring these options.

It can be debated whether percutaneous tracheostomy undertaken without bronchoscopic guidance is poor practice. The authors both feel that bronchoscopy is a useful aid when performing percutaneous tracheostomies. The authors now advocate the routine use of bronchoscopy unless there is a specific contraindication. It is unlikely that third world units will have bronchoscopes to use in this way.

Ultrasound

Ultrasonography may be used to image soft tissues around the trachea and the tracheal wall. The physics of ultrasound result in

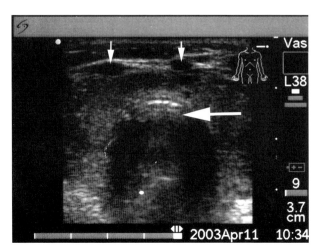

Fig. 10.5 Transverse ultrasound image of the anterior neck showing anterior jugular veins (small arrows) and acoustic shadows of trachea (large arrow): the distance from the surface of the skin to the anterior tracheal wall measures 1.5 cm.

reflection of all sound waves at a tissue/air interface, hence the inside of the air filled trachea cannot be imaged. Structures anterior and lateral to the trachea, including the thyroid, larger arteries and veins can be easily visualised (Figure 10.5).

The levels of tracheal cartilages and the downward slope of the trachea in relation to the skin as it descends into the chest can be demonstrated (Figure 10.6). The importance of the accurate identification of anterior neck structures during surgical tracheostomy has been emphasised.[6,7]

One of the authors (Henry G.W. Paw) now routinely employs ultrasound scanning of the neck before performing each percutaneous tracheostomy using the portable SonoSite 180 Plus® (Figure 10.7). As a result of being able to visualise the anatomy, some cases, which would otherwise have been referred for open surgical tracheostomy, have been successfully performed percutaneously.

Ultrasound can be particularly useful to assess the nature, size and orientation of blood vessels prior to tracheostomy. If arterial or venous pulsations or obvious veins are present at or near the proposed puncture site, useful information can be obtained about the risk to adjacent structures. The risks and benefits of an open *versus* percutaneous tracheostomy can then be made. It should not be

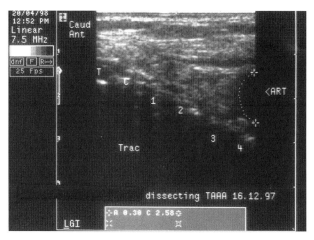

Fig. 10.6 Longitudinal ultrasound image showing the downward slope of the trachea as it descends into the chest. A large innominate artery can be seen to the right (white semicircle). T thyroid cartilage; C cricoid cartilage; first, second, third and fourth tracheal rings 1, 2, 3 and 4.

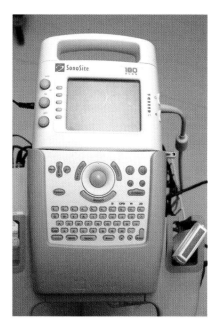

Fig. 10.7 SonoSite 180 Plus® portable ultrasound scanner.

automatically assumed that open procedures are safer in the presence of large vessels or goitre. Properly performed percutaneous techniques can cause minimal tissue disruption and bleeding. Imaging can guide needles and dilators away from at-risk structures.

Capnography

Many intensive care units (ICUs) will have access to capnography, although it has not achieved the ubiquity seen in anaesthetic practice. It can be argued that its use should be mandatory during all airway procedures in the ICU, as it is during anaesthetic and surgical practice in the operating theatre environment. However, capnography was only routinely used in 1.2% of the ICU in the most recent survey.[2] It has been used routinely when performing percutaneous tracheostomy in the unit of one of the authors' (Henry G.W. Paw) unit for over five years.

In the context of tracheostomy it is of value to confirm the following:

- Ongoing correct placement of the translaryngeal tube and pulmonary ventilation during the insertion procedure.
- Development of hypercarbia during bronchoscopy.
- Placement of the tracheostomy tube in the trachea and pulmonary ventilation.

It has also been used to confirm correct placement of the initial needle and cannula in the trachea prior to guidewire placement. It will not give any information as to the level or orientation of any such needle or cannula. It should be recognised that end tidal CO_2 values do not accurately track $PaCO_2$ values in the patient with respiratory disease.

References

1   Cooper RM. Use and safety of percutaneous tracheostomy in intensive care. *Anaesthesia* 1998; **53**: 1209–27
2   Paw HGW, Turner S. The current state of percutaneous tracheostomy in intensive care: a postal survey. *Clin Intens Care* 2002; **13**: 95–101
3   Dexter TJ. A cadaver study appraising accuracy of blind placement of percutaneous tracheostomy. *Anaesthesia* 1995; **50**: 863–4
4   Berrouschot J, Oeken J, Steiniger D. Perioperative complication following percutaneous dilatational tracheostomy. *Laryngoscope* 1997; **107**: 538–44
5   Reilly PM, Sing RF, Giberson FA, Anderson III HL, Rotondo MF, Tinkoff GH, Schwab CW. Hypercarbia during tracheostomy: a comparison of percutaneous endoscopic, percutaneous Doppler, and standard surgical tracheostomy. *Intens Care Med* 1997; **23**: 859–64
6   Bertram S, Emshoff R, Norer B. Ultrasonographic anatomy of the anterior neck: implications for tracheostomy. *J Oral Maxillofac Surg* 1995; **53**: 1420–4
7   Hatfield A, Bodenham A. Portable ultrasonic scanning of the anterior neck before percutaneous dilatational tracheostomy. *Anaesthesia* 1999; **54**: 660–3

11 Complications of Percutaneous Tracheostomy

Many of the complications of percutaneous tracheostomy (PcT) are similar to tracheostomy performed by open techniques. They may be divided into perioperative, early postoperative and late postoperative (Table 11.1). This is a useful classification, but inevitably early procedural complications may lead on to later complications. There are a large number of case series and individual case reports in the literature.[1,2]

The incidence of complications is generally low. As with other minimal access surgical techniques, however, when complications *do* occur, they can be devastating. Minor bleeding and puncture of the endotracheal (ET) tube cuff are the most common complications. A rather expensive complication is damage to the fibreoptic bronchoscope caused by the initial needle insertion. Damage to the bronchoscope can occur as the as needle can sneak in through the Murphy's eye of the ET tube, when either the ET tube is too far down the trachea or the site of needle insertion is too high up the neck (Figure 11.1).

Hypoxia and hypercapnia can be attributed to the fact that the tracheal lumen is repeatedly obstructed during the dilatation from external pressure, the presence of a bronchoscope and the dilators themselves. In children and young adults, the increased elasticity of the anterior tracheal wall may result in total compression of the tracheal lumen during the procedure. Raised intracranial pressure is due to surgical stimulus, hypoxia and hypercapnia.

There is a risk of damage to the trachea, including rupture and displacement of the tracheal rings, tear of the posterior membranous part of the trachea and tracheo-oesophageal fistula. These may be

Table 11.1 **Complications of percutaneous tracheostomy**

Perioperative	Bleeding (from veins, arteries and the thyroid gland) Puncture of the ET tube cuff Needle damage to fibreoptic bronchoscope Dislodgement of the ET tube Anaesthetic awareness
	Hypoxia Hypercapnia Increased intracranial pressure
	Damage to the trachea Damage to the oesophagus False passage of tracheostomy tube Airway obstruction due to blood clot in airway Pneumothorax
Early postoperative	Tension pneumothorax Surgical emphysema Collapsed lung Dislodgement of the tracheostomy tube Airway obstruction due to blood clot in airway
Late postoperative	Bleeding (including erosion into innominate artery/vein) Local/spreading stomal infection Subglottic stenosis Tracheal stenosis Tracheo-oesophageal fistula Persistent trachea to skin fistula Scarring and tethering of the trachea Mucus plugging (tube/airway obstruction)

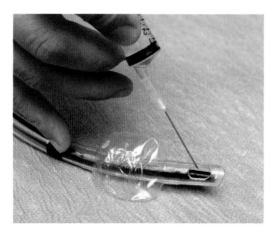

Fig. 11.1 **Needle through Murphy's eye.**

associated with bleeding, and the formation of false passages and major air leaks. The use of bronchoscopy should reduce the frequency of such complications although this has not yet been proven by clinical trial. Collapsed lung is usually a result of airway obstruction by blood clots.

Accidental dislodgement of the tracheostomy tube may be a life-threatening emergency until a tract is well established, which usually takes approximately 7 days. The initial exchange of the tracheostomy tube is generally not a problem with conventional surgical tracheostomy, even in the first few days after the procedure. However, with percutaneous techniques, immediate blind reinsertion of the tracheostomy tube is often impossible and fatal complications have been reported due to loss of the airway. The tracheostomy tube should be left in place for at least 7 days, because the stoma is dilated only, and within the first few days, the tissues will contract once a tube is removed. Over time, pressure necrosis from the tube and subsequent tissue healing around the site delineates the tract. If difficulty is encountered, the airway should be resecured by translaryngeal intubation and the tract reopened using a dilational PcT kit. Tracheal guidewire placement can be guided by bronchoscopy (see Chapter 13: Tips and Tricks).

There are now a number of publications showing that PcT is associated with a lower incidence of perioperative and early postoperative complications compared with open surgical tracheostomy. In the first prospective, randomised trial comparing PcT with open tracheostomy,[3] the original Ciaglia technique had significantly fewer complications, such as bleeding and infection (13% *versus* 46%). Similar findings were reported by others.[4] Another prospective study of 83 patients undergoing Ciaglia's PcT technique reported a lower incidence of postoperative bleeding (2.1% *versus* 13.9%; $p < 0.05$) and postoperative wound infection (0% *versus* 22.2%; $p < 0.001$) compared with open surgical tracheostomy.[5]

Controversy still surrounds the incidence of long-term complications of PcT, particularly tracheal stenosis. There are difficulties in performing long-term follow-up studies of critically ill patients who have undergone tracheostomy. These patients have a high mortality rate and lead a sedentary existence, which does not test functional tracheal patency. Many survivors may be lost to follow up. There is also no consensus as to what constitutes a significant tracheal stenosis, nor how best to diagnose it without expensive or invasive investigations.

There is currently little evidence to suggest that one technique of PcT is superior to another, as the studies performed to date are too small to detect a difference if one existed. There have been very few direct comparisons between techniques and these have tended to involve small numbers of patients studied by interested parties. The small overall percentage risk of serious complications, and high patient mortality, mean that large, expensive, multicentre studies involving hundreds of patients would be required to prove superiority of one technique over another. It is unlikely that such trials will be performed. One needs to recognise differences between results from a best operator at the top of their learning curve, compared with an average, relatively inexperienced operator. This applies equally for percutaneous or open procedures.

Early haemorrhage

Arterial or venous haemorrhage is an ever-present risk during tracheostomy. Most bleeding is minor and results from damage to the anterior jugular veins. Damage to the carotid artery and other major vessels, resulting in major haemorrhage have also been reported. The head and neck, and thyroid gland have a very rich arterial and venous blood supply. Paradoxically, the trachea itself has a rather tenuous blood supply.[6] It is unusual to see significant bleeding problems from the trachea itself.

The venous anatomy in the neck is extremely variable, and suggestions that the midline of the neck is relatively avascular are clearly untrue (Figures 11.2 and 11.3). Likewise, the arterial supply to the neck is very variable. The subclavian arteries may arise well above the clavicle and carotid arteries may cross the trachea.[7] Arteries may become tortuous and ectatic in the older patient. In addition, previous surgery in the neck may produce scarring, which pulls large vessels into the midline and tethers them to the trachea

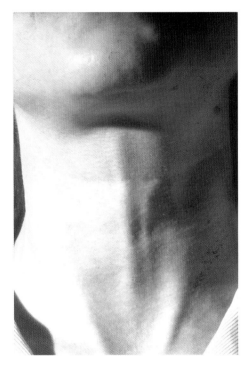

Fig. 11.2 Prominent midline veins.

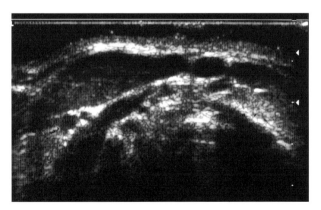

Fig. 11.3 Ultrasound of neck showing midline veins.

itself, with the potential for damage, even with the use of blunt dilators. The innominate vessels (artery and vein) cross in front of the trachea, usually behind the sternum, and are therefore vulnerable to damage both during insertion procedures and from late erosion from tube or cuff.

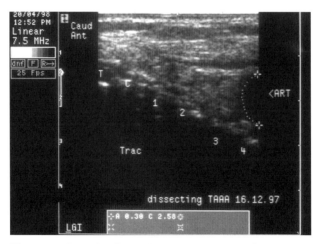

Fig. 11.4 Longitudinal ultrasound image of trachea in a man with dissecting thoracic aorta and obvious arterial pulsation above the sternum. A large innominate artery can be seen to the right (white semicircle, <ART). T: thyroid cartilage; C: cricoid cartilage; first, second, third and fourth tracheal rings are 1, 2, 3 and 4, respectively. A PcT was safely performed in theatres following discussion with cardiothoracic surgeons. Note the steep downward angle of the trachea.

Venous bleeding can usually be controlled by digital pressure or insertion of a tightly fitting tracheostomy tube or the tracheostomy dilators themselves (see Chapter 13: Tips and Tricks). Arterial bleeding from major arteries is more of a problem, and there have been a number of cases of fatal torrential haemorrhage due to tears in major arteries.[8] Such cases are commonly not recorded in the literature, but the authors are aware of a number of similar cases from medicolegal work, and discussions with clinical colleagues. The authors are also aware of similar cases following open tracheostomy procedures.

Strategies to avoid bleeding include close inspection and palpation of the neck before starting procedures. This may reveal pulsatile arterial vessels, obviously visible jugular veins or other abnormal anatomy. Ultrasound and other imaging can be used to identify arteries or veins, which are potentially at risk during procedures (Figure 11.4).

In difficult cases, it is worth discussing with surgical colleagues the optimum approach to tracheostomy. It is wrong to always consider an open procedure to be the safest option, as open procedures may leave the at-risk vessel (e.g. innominate vein) lying open within the

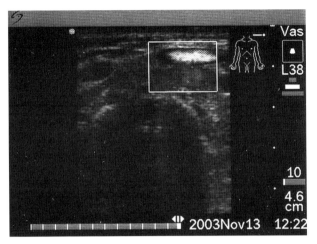

Fig. 11.5 Large 1.5 cm anterior jugular vein very close to the midline highlighted using Doppler imaging (white box). PcT was successfully inserted just off centre (avoiding the vein) by the one of the authors (Henry G.W. Paw).

tracheostomy stoma. It may be better to perform an ultrasound-guided percutaneous procedure with minimal dissection in a controlled environment in theatre. The minimum tissue dissection leaves an intact bridge of tissues between vessels and stoma. An off midline stoma may be helpful in such circumstances to avoid at-risk anatomy (Figure 11.5).

It is the authors' practice to do some blunt dissection prior to cannulating the trachea. One advantage of this is to feel for pulsatile vessels and visualise any anterior jugular veins that can then be tied off if necessary. If veins are torn during this dissection period, the situation is usually controllable, provided there is not a large hole in the trachea that then allows influx of blood into the trachea.

In the event of troublesome bleeding, urgent surgical exploration of the neck is indicated. Various manoeuvres, including putting one's finger behind the sternum and pressing on vessels, have been advocated in the literature. The percutaneous dilators can provide excellent tamponade of a bleeding stoma. Venous bleeds are usually controllable by digital pressure above and below stoma. One of the authors (Andrew R. Bodenham) has had to take a patient to theatre in this fashion in the past! In the case of a major arterial bleed, senior ear, nose and throat (ENT), vascular or cardiothoracic surgical intervention will be required very quickly to save the situation.

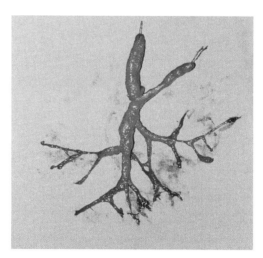

Fig. 11.6 Blood cast from the bronchial tree. This was coughed up by a patient through a tracheostomy tube. Initially appearing as a solid clot, it has been opened out, to display its branched structure, formed as a cast of the bronchial tree.

A sternotomy may be required and it is pointless to just call the junior surgical trainees, who will not have the necessary level of expertise.

Of equal concern is bleeding into the trachea. Blood will rapidly clot in the trachea and the authors have seen a number of cases of partial or total airway obstruction.[9] This may follow an obvious large bleed or occur more insidiously over a period of hours or even days due to a slow trickle of blood into the airways (Figure 11.6). Equally, blood arising from the distal airway itself can fill up the proximal airways to produce clots.

Clots arising in the major airways then may dislodge to produce total airway obstruction (Figure 11.7). A ball valve effect may occur, allowing gas into the trachea, but progressive over-expansion of the lungs due to gas trapping as the clot falls back onto the tip of the tracheal tube on expiration.

Blood clots will not pass up standard suction catheters or the suction channels of a fibreoptic scope. Large casts of the lower airway can be removed by suctioning onto the end of a fibreoptic bronchoscope and removing the bronchoscope and clot together. Alternatively, suction can be applied directly on the ET tube and the tube and clot

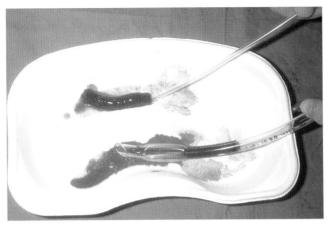

Blood clot will not pass up standard suction catheter (top), but can be suctioned into the much larger bore of an ET tube.

then removed (using a similar technique as that described for removal of aspirated meconium in the neonate). A spontaneously breathing patient may cough the clot up and out through a tracheal tube.

Late haemorrhage

Late tracheo-innominate vein/artery fistula is a feared complication of tracheostomy. A combination of erosion from the tube or cuff and local infection leads to progressive damage to the vessel wall and subsequent rupture of the vessel with potentially life-threatening haemorrhage into the airway, neck and chest. Such bleeds may be preceded by the presence of smaller warning bleeds from the stoma or trachea. Similar bleeding may occur from erosion of smaller arteries or veins in the neck due to the same mechanisms. Any bleeding should be taken seriously as it may herald massive haemorrhage later.[10]

Bleeding from smaller vessels should be controllable by surgical exploration, tying off vessels, packing the wound and digital pressure (Figure 11.8). There are reports of successful resuscitation and surgical repair following massive tracheo-innominate haemorrhage,[11] but in the authors' experience, such massive haemorrhage is usually fatal.

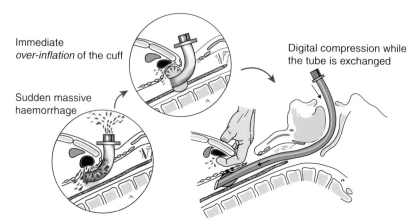

Immediate *over-inflation* of the cuff

Sudden massive haemorrhage

Digital compression while the tube is exchanged

Fig. 11.8 Mechanisms of bleeding from erosion into great vessels. Bleeding problems may be controllable by digital pressure within the stoma against the sternum. The airway should be secured early by translaryngeal intubation to prevent blood entering and obstructing the airway.

Potential avoidable causes include:

1.   Siting the skin incision or tracheal stoma too low. Traditionally, stomas are sited between the first and second or second and third tracheal rings. In the patient with a short neck and lung emphysema, it may only be feasible to site the tube at the level of the cricoid/first tracheal ring. A lower site may carry the risk of the tube lying immediately at the sternal notch in close proximity to innominate vessels. It is relevant to note that cricothyroid placement of tracheostomy tubes has been shown to be safe for longer-term patients as well as in the emergency setting.[12] Low tracheal stomas behind the sternum will provide potential difficulties when tracheostomy tubes require changing (see Chapter 13: Tips and Tricks).

2.   Insertion of a tracheostomy tube that is too short. If the stem of the tracheostomy tube is too short for the tissue tract between the skin and the trachea, then the following will occur:
     • Patient discomfort and difficulty on suctioning, as the tube tip will not lie correctly in the trachea.
     • The tension from the tissue tract will apply pressure on the external securing wings of the tracheostomy tube to produce skin necrosis and erosion of the stomal wound. With an open surgical tracheostomy stoma, the tube wings will progressively sink into the wound.

- Worse still, by the same mechanism, traction on the inflated cuff within the trachea will produce progressive necrosis of the anterior tracheal wall at the site of the tracheal stoma. The cuff may then erode through the tracheal wall into the great vessels.

There have been reports of a 'defatting' procedure during open surgical tracheostomy procedures to prevent the above scenarios, but this would not be feasible in the percutaneous techniques.[13]

3. Prevention of stomal infection. It is not clear whether tracheo-innominate fistula is more or less common after open *versus* percutaneous techniques. However, basic principles would suggest that the minimisation of tissue damage by lack of dissection and the lower infection rates associated with percutaneous techniques should make such complications less common.

Airway damage

PcT techniques rely on blunt dilators in the form of forceps or plastic dilators, which are used to force open a stoma in the tracheal wall. Such manoeuvres carry a risk of damage to the following:

- Structures in front of the trachea, e.g. the thyroid isthmus and blood vessels.
- The tracheal wall itself, either the anterior, lateral or posterior membranous sections.
- Related structures, e.g. the oesophagus.

Bleeding has been covered in the previous section. The anterior and side walls of the trachea may get torn, cartilages may fracture and be pushed into the tracheal lumen. Any such distortion may then scar and produce stenosis.[14]

The membranous part of the trachea posteriorly is particularly susceptible to damage. Studies have suggested that damage, usually minor, is far more common than realised.[15] Studies have been performed on sheep showing that cartilage damage and mucosal tears on the anterior and posterior wall of the trachea are very common, with minor damage occurring in all cases.[16] Similar findings have been reported in cadaver studies.[17] The relevance of such findings to the comparative incidence of complications, like tracheal stenosis between open and percutaneous techniques, is unknown.

PcT has never gained popularity in children, in part due to fears of tracheal complications like stenosis in an already narrow structure. The compliant nature of a child's trachea may give further problems during insertion techniques.[18]

In most cases of minor tracheal damage, there are no clinical sequelae. Larger tears may result in an air leak, air emphysema, pneumothorax and an oesophageal tear with mediastinitis. Such tears may be managed either conservatively by passage of a long stem adjustable flange tracheostomy tube, or an uncut long translaryngeal ET tube, past the tear to allow natural healing over time. Bronchoscopic verification of tube positioning is desirable in such cases. Alternatively, a surgical repair of the trachea/oesophagus may be undertaken by open or endoscopic techniques. In the event of such damage, the situation should be discussed with senior thoracic or ENT surgical colleagues. A decision regarding surgical or conservative management should be made after careful consideration of the condition of the patient and their fitness for a major surgical and anaesthetic intervention. In the authors' own units, cases have been managed successfully with both approaches.

Damage to the trachea can be minimised by careful attention to detail and operator experience. Flexible soft dilators and tubes with beveled ends should be used whenever possible and excessive forces avoided. Excessively large-bore tubes should be avoided. Correct positioning of guidewires and dilators can be established using procedural bronchoscopy. However, it should be appreciated that once larger dilators are inserted and during placement of the tracheostomy tube itself, there is considerable distortion of the images. Bronchoscopy at this stage does not give adequate visualisation to guarantee that damage to the airway is not occurring. Equally, tears lying within the area of the tracheostomy tube will not be easily visible without tube withdrawal or removal. Further damage may result from difficult or traumatic tracheostomy tube changes later in the course of the patient's illness.

There has been discussion regarding the merits of the different dilators, but to date, no adequate trials have definitively shown that one technique is superior to another in this respect.

Air leaks/pneumothorax

Surgical emphysema and pneumothorax are well-recognised problems following PcT (Figures 11.9 and 11.10). Air leaks may arise from pre-existing lung pathology. Alternatively, the procedure may cause an air leak via the following mechanisms.

- Air leak from the trachea during the procedure, in particular if a finger is used to block air leakage from the stoma.
- Positive pressure ventilation via a misplaced tracheostomy tube in a paratracheal position will cause massive air emphysema which may track down into the chest and drain into on or both pleural spaces to produce a tension pneumothorax.
- Tears of the tracheal wall, ± oesophageal tear may produce similar problems.
- Needle damage to the lung apex is also possible.

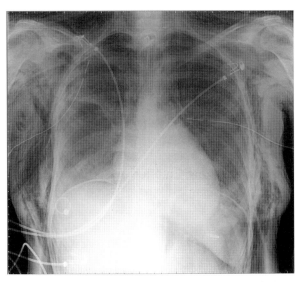

Fig. 11.9 Widespread surgical emphysema following PcT. There is air above and below the diaphragm and bilateral pneumothoraces have been drained.

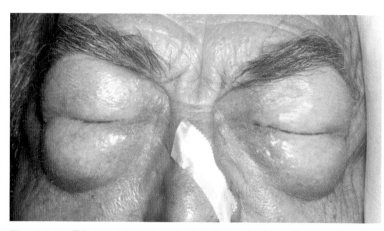

Fig. 11.10 Bilateral facial and orbital surgical emphysema following PcT. Such emphysema may just spread up one side of the face.

- Air leaks from the fenestrations of speaking tubes have also been observed when the fenestrations lie within the stoma rather than in the tracheal lumen.

Small amounts of air emphysema will usually settle over time but it should be appreciated that any air leak may herald a significant pneumothorax or airway trauma. The need for X-ray imaging or further endoscopic examination should be carefully considered.[19]

Tube dislodgement/obstruction

Tracheostomy tubes may be incorrectly inserted in a paratracheal position both on initial insertion or subsequent tube change. Alternatively, the tip of the tube but not the cuff may lie within the trachea. The end orifice of tubes may lie against the back or sidewall of the trachea, rather than facing directly downwards to produce increased resistance or obstruction.[20]

This may not be noticed if the patient is breathing spontaneously, but complications of positive pressure ventilation will lead to development of air emphysema, which may then spread down into the mediastinum to produce a tension pneumothorax. The patient will become increasingly hypoxic and hypercarbic. Similar mechanisms may occur later if the tracheostomy tube becomes dislodged and reinsertion proves difficult.

Accidental dislodgement of tracheostomy tube may be a life-threatening emergency until a tract is well established, which usually takes approximately 7 days. Such dislodgement is thought to be less common with PcT than open procedures, due to the snug fit of tubes. The initial exchange of the tracheostomy tube is generally not a problem with conventional surgical tracheostomy, even in the first few days after the procedure. However, with percutaneous techniques, immediate reinsertion of the tracheal cannula is virtually impossible and fatal complications have been reported. Resecure the airway with translaryngeal intubation. With PcT, the original tracheostomy tube should be left in place for at least 7 days, because the stoma is dilated only, and within the first few days, the tissue will contract when tubes are removed.

Tracheal stenosis

Following tracheostomy, most patients will develop some degree of tracheal scarring, granuloma formations and narrowing around the site of the tracheal stoma, and where the cuff has pressed on the trachea. A small percentage will go on to develop progressive scarring and narrowing of the trachea, and develop symptomatic stenosis. It should be appreciated that many lesser stenoses are asymptomatic, particularly in a sedentary patient. It is not clear why some patients develop such severe stenosis. It is a common belief that the young male patient with a brain injury may be particularly at risk (Figure 11.11).

Stenoses may affect a short or longer segment of trachea (Figure 11.12). There is no consensus as to what is significant tracheal stenosis, and how best to diagnose it (Figure 11.13). Studies based solely on symptomatology grossly underestimate the incidence of stenotic lesions. It is estimated that the tracheal lumen of an adult needs to be reduced by up to 75% of its diameter before symptoms are noted. However, clinically significant tracheal stenosis appears to be rare after PcT. Using nasendoscopy, Law *et al.*[21] followed 41 intensive care survivors who had previously undergone a Ciaglia PcT, for at least 6 months after decannulation and reported that all 41 patients were asymptomatic, despite four patients (10%) having a significant (>10%) tracheal stenosis. They also commented that

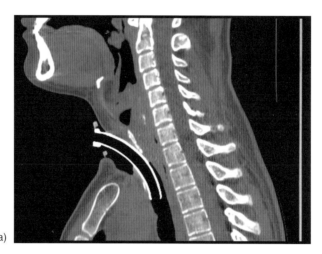

(a)

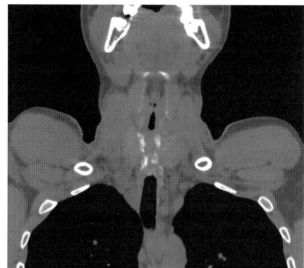

(b)

Fig. 11.11 (a and b) Severe tracheal stenosis in a young man ventilated for head injury using translaryngeal intubation and a PcT. Sagittal and coronal reconstructed CT images show complete obliteration of the tracheal lumen from just below the larynx down the tracheostomy stoma. The larynx is also thickened and damaged. There is extensive scar tissue with calcification. Such lesions produce major difficulties for tracheal reconstructive surgery.

flow-volume loops were of limited value in diagnosing tracheal stenosis in these patients.

Other studies have also shown the incidence of symptomatic tracheal stenosis to be reassuringly small following PcT. The other issue is whether the different techniques of PcT are associated with a different

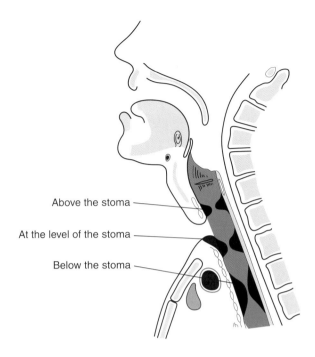

Above the stoma

At the level of the stoma

Below the stoma

Fig. 11.12 Tracheal damage and stenosis may occur at one or more sites after tracheostomy.

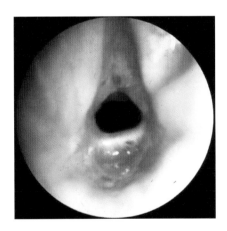

Fig. 11.13 Subglottic tracheal stenosis following translaryngeal intubation.

incidence of tracheal stenosis. A prospective, randomised study comparing the Ciaglia technique and Griggs' Portex technique[22] followed 80 patients for 9 months and found no clinically relevant tracheal stenosis. Studies looking at the incidence of tracheal stenosis following open surgical tracheostomy,[23] however, have reported much higher incidence compared with PcT. These studies are, however, old and the incidence is probably lower since the introduction of softer tubes with high-volume low-pressure cuffs. Clearly, there is a need for prospective, randomised trials to compare long-term outcome after the percutaneous techniques and open surgical tracheostomy. These studies will require large numbers of patients.

Mechanisms of tracheal damage

Various mechanisms are likely to play a part in causing damage. Traumatic insertion or reinsertion of ET or tracheostomy tubes, and the use of large dilators, cause direct trauma, particularly if tracheal rings are pushed inwards. The repeated passage of suction catheters to remove secretions may damage the tracheal mucosa. The duration of insult is important; damage is likely to worsen over time. Damage can occur after surprisingly short periods of tracheal intubation.

Ischaemic necrosis may occur in the tracheal mucosa cartilages from the pressure of the tube itself or the inflated cuff (Figure 11.14). Exposed cartilages may become infected and collapse. The tracheal blood supply is relatively poor, even in health. Critical illness or vasopressor drugs may further reduce the perfusion of the trachea and its mucosa. It is probable that in most cases a number of these factors interact to produce progressive destruction of the trachea, which then heals with scarring.

The formation of granulation tissue at the site of the stoma seems to be of importance (Figure 11.15). It has been suggested that regular changing of tracheostomy tubes might be of value to slow the formation of granulomas.[24]

It must be appreciated that most patients undergoing PcT will already have had a variable duration of translaryngeal intubation with the potential for airway damage to have occurred before tracheostomy (Figure 11.13). The tracheostomy procedure may then add to existing damage or cause problems in its own right. Unless serial endoscopy is carried out it will be impossible to know which procedure or interventions are responsible.[23,25,26]

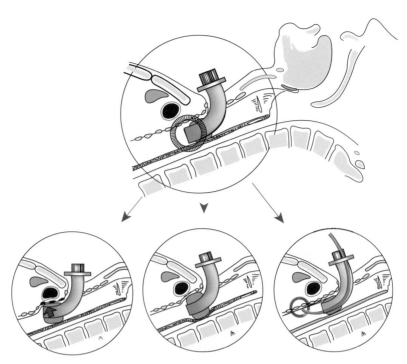

Fig. 11.14 Diagrammatic representation of mechanisms of injury for tracheal damage following tracheostomy.

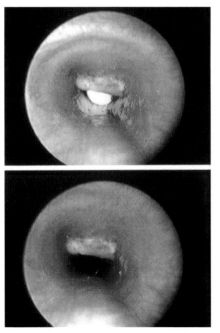

Fig. 11.15 An adolescent after PcT. A cartilage ring has been pushed inwards and a granuloma formed. The granuloma required laser resection.

The role of cuff pressure

Although the inflated cuff is an obvious culprit, other mechanisms may contribute to the damage as discussed previously in this chapter. In simple terms, the presence of the tube and its inflated cuff causes pressure necrosis of the mucosa (inner lining of the trachea), muscle layers and cartilages in the trachea. Over time, the injured area heals with scarring, which may contract to result in a narrowing or stenosis. Some degree of mucosal injury is inevitable in every case but very few patients develop severe stenosis. It is not understood why some patients develop such a severe scarring whilst the majority do not. The true incidence of such problems is not known and in many patients, the picture is complicated by the double insult of translaryngeal intubation followed by tracheostomy.

The cuff provides two main functions:

1. To provide a seal to enable positive pressure ventilation of the lung without a significant air leak. The higher the pressures required to ventilate the lung the higher the pressure required in the cuff to provide a seal. High pressures in the breathing circuit can further raise the pressure in the cuff by back pressure from the trachea.[27]
2. To provide a seal to prevent aspiration of secretions into the trachea (e.g. stomach contents, bile and nasopharyngeal secretions).

Currently in the UK, most intensive care units (ICUs) do not measure cuff pressures routinely.[28] The measurement of pressures in the cuff has its limitations. It is not a direct measure of the applied pressure to the mucosa. Most units rely on inflating the cuff so that there is no leak (or minimum leak) with positive pressure ventilation. If pressures *are* measured, current recommendations are to keep the pressure below 25–30 mmHg, whenever possible. Over-inflation of cuffs cannot be seen on X-rays unless gross damage occurs with disruption of the structure of the trachea.

The numerous studies that have been performed in this area have failed to find a perfect solution to the problem despite the invention of numerous different tubes, cuffs, measurement devices and pressure-relieving valves. Clinical problems do seem to have reduced since the 1960–1970s with the advent of safer, softer biocompatible tubes with high-volume low-pressure cuffs. It should be appreciated that profile cuffs will not perform adequately if the tracheal tube is too small for the individual patient's trachea. Unfortunately, there is no ideal size tube for an individual patient and no easy bedside test to measure tracheal diameter to aid choice of tube size.

Management of the patient with tracheal stenosis

Patients with significant tracheal stenosis (Figure 11.16) will typically present with signs of airway obstruction, stridor and respiratory insufficiency with slow weaning from assisted ventilation. A diagnosis is made on endoscopy and other investigations like computed tomography (CT) and magnetic resonance imaging (MRI).[29]

Patients should be referred to a thoracic or ENT surgeon who has a specialised interest in this esoteric field. In the symptomatic patient, relief can be obtained by serial dilation of the stenosis or tracheal stent placement (Figure 11.17). Alternatively, direct surgical repair can be performed with resection of the stenotic segments and tracheal end-to-end anastomosis. Such surgery is hazardous and many such

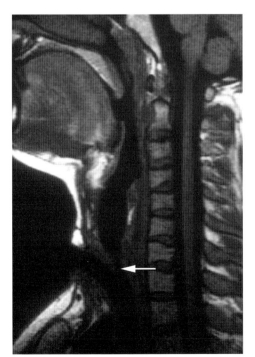

Fig. 11.16 A sagittal section MRI showing tracheal stenosis following open surgical tracheostomy. A narrow segment of the trachea is stenosed (white arrow) immediately above the stoma. A short section of narrowing like this is amenable to successful surgical resection and tracheal end-to-end anastomosis.

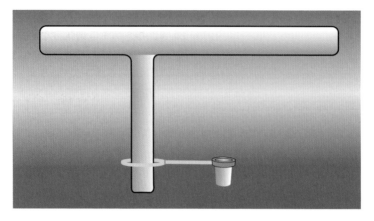

Fig. 11.17
T tube stent.

patients will regrettably end up requiring long-term tracheostomy. Surgery is hindered by the fact that there is to date no satisfactory natural or artificial prosthetic material that provides rigidity to facilitate repairs of the trachea.[30]

Tracheo-oesophageal fistula

Tracheo-oesophageal fistula may occur from a tear in the membranous part of the trachea extending into the oesophagus. Alternatively, over-inflation of tracheal cuffs can produce progressive erosion of the trachea into the oesophagus (Figure 11.18). A surgical repair is required, but is fraught with problems.[31]

Infection

Tracheostomy stomas inevitably become colonised with organisms from the trachea, bronchi and oropharynx. It used to be proposed that tracheostomy increased the risk of nosocomial pneumonia, though this is now not thought to be the case. More severe spreading cellulitis can occur around the stoma itself. This used to be a relatively common feature following open tracheostomies in the critically ill patient. Prior to the advent of PcT, the authors were aware and saw a number of deaths in ICUs from this complication, as a terminal event to critical illness. Streptococcus was the most common organism isolated. The advent of PcT has led to a dramatic reduction in the incidence of such local infectious

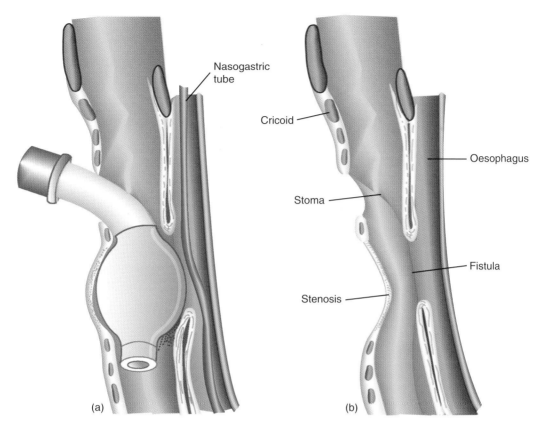

Fig. 11.18 Origin and anatomy of postintubation tracheoesophageal fistula. Lateral diagrams of the trachea and oesophagus. (a) The overdistended cuff has injured the trachea circumferentially. The 'party wall' posteriorly has become devascularized and has necrosed by being pinched between the cuff and a firm nasogastric tube in the oesophagus. (b) The fistula is usually below the stoma, at the level of the balloon cuff. (Redrawn from Grillo HC (Ed). *Surgery of the Trachea and Bronchi*. 2004: BC Decker Inc; Hamilton, Ontario.)

complications (see Chapter 6: Advantages of Percutaneous *versus* Open Surgical Tracheostomy). The probable explanation for this reduced infection is the minimal dissection used in PcT, which limits tissue damage in and around the trachea. However, such infections do still occur rarely (Figures 11.19 and 11.20).

Mucus plugging and airway obstruction

Immediately following a PcT, a collapsed lung is usually due to obstruction by blood clots. Later problems are usually due to mucus

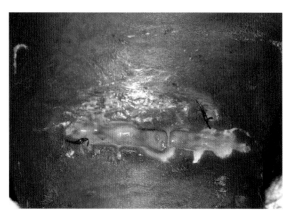

Fig. 11.19 Tracheal stoma infection following open surgical tracheostomy.

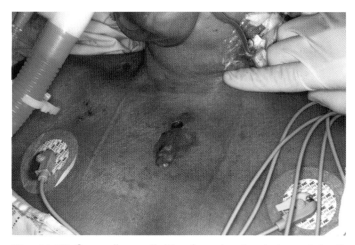

Fig. 11.20 Spreading cellulites from tracheal stoma infection following a rather low PcT. Methicillin-resistant *Staphylococcus aureus* (MRSA) was isolated from the wound and the infection successfully managed with vancomycin antibiotic therapy.

plugging and progressive airway obstruction usually due to excessive secretions. Inadequate suctioning, physiotherapy or humidification will exacerbate the situation. Mucus plugs may block the tracheostomy tube itself or break free and produce total airway obstruction within the trachea. Hence, a change of tracheostomy tube or inner liner may not help in the latter situation. Such problems are a major concern in patients who are discharged from specialist areas into general ward areas where care may be inadequate.[32]

Long-term tracheal to skin fistula

Tracheostomy stomas are usually left to granulate spontaneously after decannulation. In well-formed tracts, the mucosal surfaces may not heal completely, leaving a small mucous fistula between trachea and skin. This may periodically discharge mucus or pus. Such tracts, if troublesome, require surgical excision and closure. Alternatively, the scar may heal, with tethering, to produce deformity or difficulty in swallowing. Again, surgical excision and closure is required.

References

1   Walz MK, *et al.* Percutaneous dilatational tracheostomy – early results and long-term outcome of 326 critically ill patients. *Intens Care Med* 1998; **24**: 685–90
2   Rosenbower TJ, Morris Jr JA, Eddy VA, Ries WR. The long-term complications of percutaneous dilatational tracheostomy. *Am Surg* 1998; **64**: 82–6
3   Hazard P, Jones C, Benitone J. Comparative trial of standard operative tracheostomy with percutaneous tracheostomy. *Crit Care Med* 1991; **19**: 1018–24
4   Friedman Y, Fildes J, Mizock B, Samuel J, Patel S, Appavu S, Roberts R. Comparison of percutaneous and surgical tracheostomies. *Chest* 1996; **110**: 480–5
5   Stoeckli SJ, Breitbach T, Schmid S. A clinical and histologic comparison of a percutaneous dilatational versus conventional surgical tracheostomy. *Laryngoscope* 1997; **107**: 1643–6
6   Allen MS. Surgical anatomy of the trachea. *Chest Surg Clin North Am* 2003; **13**: 191–9
7   Farmery AD, Shlugman D, Anslow P. How high do the subclavian arteries ascend into the neck? A population study using magnetic resonance imaging. *Br J Anaesth* 2003; **90**: 452–6
8   Shlugman D, Satya-Krishna R, Loh L. Acute fatal haemorrhage during percutaneous dilatational tracheostomy. *Br J Anaesth* 2003; **90**: 517–20
9   Bodenham A. Removal of obstructing blood clot from the lower airway: an alternative suction technique. *Anaesthesia* 2002; **57**: 40–43
10 Bernard SA, Jones BM, Shearer WA. Percutaneous dilatational tracheostomy complicated by delayed life-threatening haemorrhage. *Aust New Zeal J Surg* 1992; **62**: 152–3
11 Allan JS, Wright CD. Tracheoinnominate fistula: diagnosis and management. *Chest Surg Clin North Am* 2003; **13**: 331–41
12 Brantigan CO, Grow Sr JB. Subglottic stenosis after cricothyroidotomy. *Surgery* 1982; **91**: 217–21
13 Gross ND, Cohen JI, Andersen PE. 'Defatting' tracheotomy in morbidly obese patients. *Laryngoscope* 2002; **112**: 1940–44
14 Walz MK, Schmidt U. Tracheal lesion caused by percutaneous dilatational tracheostomy – a clinico-pathological study. *Intens Care Med* 1999; **25**: 102–5
15 Trottier SJ, Hazard PB, Sakabu SA, Levine JH, Troop BR, Thompson JA, McNary R. Posterior tracheal wall perforation during percutaneous dilational tracheostomy: an investigation into its mechanism and prevention. *Chest* 1999; **115**: 1383–9

16 Nickells JS, Dahlstrom JE, Bidstrup H, Dobbinson TL. Acute tracheal trauma in sheep caused by percutaneous tracheostomy. *Anaesth Intens Care* 2002; **30**: 619–23

17 Hotchkiss KS, McCaffrey JC. Laryngotracheal injury after percutaneous dilational tracheostomy in cadaver specimens. *Laryngoscope* 2003; **113**: 16–20

18 Scott CJ, Darowski M, Crabbe DC. Complications of percutaneous dilational tracheostomy in children. *Anaesthesia* 1998; **53**: 477–80

19 Kaylie DM, Wax MK. Massive subcutaneous emphysema following percutaneous tracheostomy. *Am J Otolaryngol* 2002; **23**: 300–2

20 Trottier SJ, Ritter S, Lakshmanan R, Sakabu SA, Troop BR. Percutaneous tracheostomy tube obstruction. *Chest* 2002; **122**: 1377–81

21 Law RC, Carney S, Manara AR. Long-term outcome after percutaneous dilatational tracheostomy. Endoscopic and spirometry findings. *Anaesthesia* 1997; **52**: 51–6

22 Ambesh SP, Kaushik S. Percutaneous dilatatinal tracheostomy: the Ciaglia method *versus* the Rapitrach method. *Anesth Analg* 1998; **87**: 556–61

23 Stauffer JL, Olson DE, Petty TL. Complications and consequences of endotracheal intubation and tracheostomy: a prospective study of 150 critically ill adult patients. *Am J Med* 1981; **70**: 65–76

24 Yaremchuk K. Regular tracheostomy tube changes to prevent the formation of granulation tissue. *Laryngoscope* 2003; **113**: 1–10

25 Bishop MJ, Weymuller Jr EA, Fink BR. Laryngeal effects of prolonged intubation. *Anesth Analg* 1984; **63**: 335–42

26 Chagnon FP, Mulder DS. Laryngotracheal trauma. *Chest Surg Clin North Am* 1996; **6**: 733–48

27 Guyton DC, Barlow MR, Besselievre TR. Influence of airway pressure on minimum occlusive endotracheal tube cuff pressure. *Crit Care Med* 1997; **25**: 91–4

28 Vyas D, Inweregbu K, Pittard A. Measurement of tracheal tube cuff pressure in critical care. *Anaesthesia* 2002; **57**: 275–7

29 Weber AL. Radiologic evaluation of the trachea. *Chest Surg Clin North Am* 1996; **6**: 637–73

30 Couraud L, Jougon JB, Ballester M. Techniques of management of subglottic stenoses with glottic and supraglottic problems. *Chest Surg Clin North Am* 1996; **6**: 791–809

31 Dartevelle P, Macchiarini P. Management of acquired tracheoesophageal fistula. *Chest Surg Clin North Am* 1996; **6**: 819–36

32 Heafield S, Rogers M, Karnik A. Tracheostomy management in ordinary wards. *Hosp Med* 1999; **60**: 261–2

Further reading

Grillo HC. *Surgery of the Trachea and Bronchi*, 2004: BC Decker; Hamilton, Ontario

Aftercare, Decannulation and Follow-up

Timely percutaneous tracheostomy has revolutionised airway management in the intensive care unit (ICU), making weaning and discharge much easier for the sicker patient. However, the advantages to the patient and ICU come at a price. Tracheostomy care is generally well understood by medical staff, nurses and physiotherapists in the intensive care, theatre and specialised ward environments, but there are major deficiencies in knowledge outside these more specialist areas. There are therefore major risks in sending patients with a tracheostomy to a general ward, staffed by relatively inexperienced staff that will not be confident or capable of looking after such patients. Over the years, repeated problems with inadequate tracheostomy care in the general ward situation have been observed.

Without adequate humidification, physiotherapy and suction, tracheostomy tubes rapidly get blocked with thick secretions, which, if untreated, will lead to airway obstruction and eventually respiratory and cardiac arrest. Untrained attending staff will not be confident in changing tracheostomy tubes, unblocking tubes or ventilating the patient through a tracheostomy tube in an emergency situation. The authors are aware of many patients who have come to harm in such situations, where they have suffered a respiratory arrest due to tracheostomy tube blockage and attending staff has been unable to salvage the situation. Airway obstruction will produce progressively worse hypoxia, with subsequent respiratory and then cardiac arrest. Futile attempts to resuscitate a patient by bag and facemask ventilation have been attempted in the presence of a blocked cuffed tracheostomy tube *in situ*. Staff may fail to appreciate that there is a removable inner liner in the tracheostomy tube. There are a number of high profile court cases in progress in the UK at the present time relating to this scenario, where patients have either died or been left in a persistent vegetative state due to hypoxic cardiac arrest.

Referring specialties and intensive care staff should share the responsibility of organising and providing appropriate aftercare for patients with a tracheostomy tube *in situ*, who leave the ICU/HDU for lower dependency areas. The authors attempt to place all patients with a tracheostomy into areas where the staff are familiar with the care of such patients (e.g. ICU; HDU; ENT and maxillofacial wards). The unit of one of the authors' (Henry G.W. Paw) has produced guidelines in relation to tracheostomy care and a training package. The recent introduction of 'outreach', available 24 h a day, has also contributed to the care of these patients on the general wards:

To ensure the safety of the patient with a tracheostomy, there are certain essential equipment which must remain with the patient at all times, including during transfers to the X-ray department and theatre (Box 12.1).

Box 12.1 Essential equipment

- Tracheostomy tube – same size plus one size smaller
- Tracheal dilators
- 10 ml syringe
- Suction unit, catheters and gloves
- Resuscitation bag (including self-inflating bag and tubing)
- Equipment for translaryngeal intubation if the patient is dependent on assisted ventilation

---

Ward staff need to understand the processes required for tracheostomy care and there are useful resources available on websites and distributed by companies involved with tracheostomy care. Staff should be competent enough to recognise and change blocked or dislodged tubes, and to perform resuscitation manoeuvres such as assisted ventilation through the tracheostomy tube. The various components in the care of the tracheostomy patient are listed in Box 12.2.

- Speech/communication with a tracheostomy
- Humidification
- Physiotherapy
- Suctioning
- Cuff inflation
- Tracheostomy stoma care
- Assessment of bulbar competence
- Decannulation techniques
- Tube changes
- Recognition and management of the blocked/misplaced tube
- Follow-up

The purpose of communication for the critically ill patient is to help them to maintain their identity, as well as their psychological and social integrity. The psychological status of the ICU patient must be considered, as they may be unable to speak or communicate and will often be very frightened in the ICU environment.

Whilst the tracheostomy patient remains ventilator dependent, there may be insufficient airflow through the vocal cords for them to speak. The patient should be reassured that their voice will return once the tube is removed or changed to a fenestrated speaking tube. Alternative means of communication (e.g. alphabet boards, picture boards, phrase books or writing) should be used in the meantime. There are various devices and aids for communication discussed elsewhere in this book (page 69).

The normal functions of the nose are to warm, filter and humidify the inspired air. A tracheostomy tube will bypass these natural mechanisms and the administration of dry gases will lead to poor function of the ciliated epithelial cells in the trachea. Failure to humidify the inspired gas will result in thick and inadequately cleared secretions, leading to tube occlusion and pulmonary collapse/consolidation.

The inspired air can be humidified by placing a heat moisture exchange (HME) filter or other humidifier system into the breathing circuit. In practice, most ICUs and acute care units use hot water humidification systems in the acute phase of patient care.

Assessment of bulbar competence

The presence of bulbar problems should be anticipated in the presence of brain injury, cranial nerve palsies and other neuromuscular dysfunction. The clinical presence of aspiration of gastrointestinal (GI) contents or tube feeds via the tracheostomy suggests that passive regurgitation is recurring.

The presence of a tracheostomy tube can impair the act of swallowing in several ways:

1. Reduced antero-superior movement of the larynx.
2. Reduced laryngeal closure.
3. Compression of the oesophagus by an over-inflated tracheostomy tube cuff.
4. Loss of co-ordination of the glottic closure response.
5. Reduced laryngeal sensitivity.

Neurological injury, poor conscious level or poor cough and motor function may render a patient unable to protect their airway or cough adequately to remove secretions or other aspirated material from the trachea. There is no consensus as to the ideal way to assess such functions. The patient can be asked to swallow a fluid/foodstuff with added dye (e.g. ribena drink – see Appendix 3) and the trachea is then suctioned to look for evidence of aspirated material. The value of such tests *versus* clinical observations to look for aspirated feed or a trial cuff deflation or decannulation is debatable. Some units rely on interpretation of such observations by speech therapists; other units have no speech therapy input.

Suctioning

The frequency of suctioning is dependent on the individual patient's need and requires individual assessment and constant re-assessment.

If the patient is significantly oxygen dependent, they should be pre-oxygenated with 100% FiO_2 for at least 3 min prior to suctioning. The suction catheter should be inserted with the suction off to avoid trauma. The catheter should then be inserted until the patient coughs and should go no further than the carina. The tip of the catheter should then be withdrawn by approximately 0.5 cm and continuous suction applied as the catheter is slowly withdrawn. Suction should not exceed 10 s, as prolonged suction may lead to hypoxia and the lowest possible vacuum pressure should be used to reduce complications. The vacuum pressure should be no more than 20 kPa. High negative pressure can cause mucosal trauma and atelectasis. Thick, tenacious sputum may require a larger suction catheter (up to 16 FG) and a small amount (2 ml) of sterile 0.9% saline to aid clearance by initiating a cough and loosening secretion. A mucolytic agent, such as acetylcysteine (nebulised) may help to reduce the viscosity of the sputum.

A closed-system, multiple-use ('in-line') suction unit can be used for patients on assisted ventilation. This is useful in a patient who is highly oxygen/positive end expiratory pressure (PEEP) dependent with copious sputum. It also has the advantage of preventing the escape of infected sputum into the ICU environment.

When a patient is ready for decannulation of the tracheostomy tube, secretions that may have collected above the cuff, will on cuff deflation enter the bronchus if the patient has an inadequate cough. These can be removed by using a synchronised suction/cuff deflation technique, which requires two personnel (Box 12.3), or by the use of specialised tubes with an additional suction channel.

Box 12.3 Synchronised suction/cuff deflation technique prior to decannulation

- Before deflating the cuff, suction gently with a 12–16 FG suction catheter (not a Yankauer) in the oropharynx
- Pass a new sterile suction catheter into the tracheostomy tube approximately 0.5 cm longer than the tracheostomy tube tip
- Apply suction as the cuff is deflated gradually in 0.5 ml increments allowing the secretions to be removed as they pass down the gradually deflating cuff

Cuff inflation

When inflating the cuff, the minimum volume should be used to prevent air leaks. A 10 ml syringe is used to gradually inflate the cuff at 0.5 ml increments. A stethoscope is placed just below the thyroid cartilage to listen for any air leaks. Normal hearing should not be relied upon – a stethoscope is required for accuracy. Estimation of cuff pressure by fingertip pressure on the external pilot balloon is inaccurate. There are commercially available devices to monitor such pressures (see page 65).

Tracheostomy stoma care

The aim is to keep the stoma clean and dry, reducing the risk of skin irritation and infection. Secretions may pool above the tracheostomy tube cuff and escape through the stoma site leading to skin maceration and excoriation. These in turn may act as a growth medium for microbes and impair stoma wound healing.

A slim and absorbent dressing with a pre-cut central keyhole (e.g. Lyofoam® or Allevyn®) are suitable for use as a tracheostomy dressing. The smooth, shiny side should be placed in contact with the skin. These hydrophilic, polyurethane foam dressings are preferable as they are designed to absorb moisture away from the skin interface, reducing skin maceration. The tracheal tube tie and dressing should be changed at least every 24 h, and earlier if wet or soiled. The frequency of dressing change is dependent on the amount of secretion oozing around the stoma and should be reviewed every 8 h.

Changing a tracheostomy tube

It is recommended that tracheostomy tubes without an inner cannula should be changed every 10–14 days to avoid the risk of occlusion with dried secretions. A tracheostomy with an inner cannula may remain for 30 days. Early signs of potential tracheostomy tube occlusion include respiratory distress or difficulty in passing a suction catheter.

The first change should be performed by medical personnel that are competent in airway management. This is because the stoma and track may not be well formed and can close up rapidly, requiring translaryngeal intubation.

The patient should be nil by mouth for 4–6 h before a tube change. The nasogastric (NG) tube, if present, should be aspirated just before the procedure. The patient should be pre-oxygenated with 100% oxygen if oxygen-dependent and oxygen-saturation levels are monitored. The patient should be positioned in a semi-recumbent position with the neck extended. The cuff should be checked on the new tube by inflating it and rolling back the cuff as it is deflated fully (see Chapter 13: Tips and Tricks). Both the tracheostomy tube and cuff should be lubricated. Using the synchronised suction/cuff deflation technique (Box 12.3), the second helper should slowly deflate the cuff and remove the old tracheostomy tube. The new tube can then be inserted in an inward and downward motion. The obturator should then be removed immediately and auscultation for equal, bilateral air entry performed. The cuff should be inflated with the minimum volume required to prevent air leaks.

Decannulation and follow-up

Just as there are arguments in relation to the timing of tracheostomy formation, there are arguments about when patients should be decannulated. In theory, patients should not be decannulated until it is established that they have adequate respiratory drive, a good cough and protection of their airway by intact upper airway reflexes. It is difficult to measure any of these functions objectively. The ability to breathe without tiring and adequate oxygenation are relatively easy to establish by a trial of weaning onto a continuous positive airway pressure (CPAP) circuit or T-piece with an appropriate low humidified source of oxygen. It is more difficult to assess the patient's ability to cough adequately and clear secretions to protect their airway. There is no objective measure of cough function, but if the patient is able to physically cough secretions out of their tracheostomy tube, it is regarded as a good sign. Equally, a general assessment of the motor power elsewhere in the body will give useful information. The profoundly weak patient who cannot sit or move unaided, with a poor cough and profuse thick secretions is unlikely to be successfully decannulated longer term. Conscious level is also an important component.

Obviously, there are great psychological advantages to the patient in being able to speak and communicate. Consideration should be given to changing to uncuffed fenestrated tubes with inner liners to aid such functions. Equally, the presence of an inflated tube cuff may make swallowing difficult. A trial of cuff deflation may be useful if not contraindicated for other reasons.

It is important to assess the patient's respiratory drive, ability to cough and general muscle and bulbar function at the bedside. If this appears promising, decannulation of the patient can be considered. An alternative method is to deflate the cuff and spigot the tracheostomy tube, and observe the patient for a number of hours. In either case, subsequent decannulation should not be a problem, provided the tracheostomy stoma is well formed. The tube can be removed, the patient's trachea sucked out, and if the patient does not manage well in the subsequent hours, the tracheostomy tube can be reinserted.

It should be appreciated that in the convalescent period, the tracheostomy tube may do more harm than good. The physical presence of a tube bypasses the normal physiological functions of the upper airway in warming, humidification and filtering of air. The patient with improving muscle power and intact bulbar function will produce a more effective cough after decannulation, when they can build up a high pressure against a closed glottis, and then open the cords to achieve a strong cough. For these reasons, tracheostomy tubes should be removed, where possible, sooner rather than later.

Following decannulation, most tracheostomy stomas are allowed to granulate without suturing. Most are colonised with respiratory pathogens but will heal quickly to achieve a functional seal within 2–3 days. Such partially healed wounds can be quickly reopened with an artery forceps in the first few weeks after closure if necessary. Occasionally, tracheostomy wounds will require secondary surgical revision due to scarring, tethering of the trachea and occasional sinus formation where an epithelialised tract remains between the trachea and the skin surface. Such tracts may persist in the longer term to periodically discharge mucus or pus.

The most feared complication is tracheal stenosis, which may present after decannulation as respiratory insufficiency or stridor. It is not clear how quickly such stenoses may develop. They are seen clinically in some patients early on in their clinical course and present only following decannulation. Alternatively, they may present weeks or months later. Some writers have suggested that patients should be routinely investigated by endoscopy following tracheal decannulation. This is probably impractical, as this would need to be repeated on a regular basis for some weeks or months after decannulation. Equally, basic radiological imaging is not a practical solution, as computed tomography (CT) or magnetic resonance imaging (MRI) is required to show stenotic lesions of the trachea. Any such problems need to be referred on to ENT or thoracic surgeons with a particular interest in this area (see Chapter 11: Complications of Percutaneous Tracheostomy).

Further reading

1 Docherty B, Bench S. Tracheostomy management for patients in general ward settings. *Profess Nurse* 2002; **18**: 100–4
2 Heafield S, Rogers M, Karnik A. Tracheostomy management in ordinary wards. *Hosp Med* 1999; **60**: 261–2

Tips and Tricks

Needle angulation

Following identification of the surface landmarks, some operators angle the needle caudad in an attempt to ensure the guidewire goes caudad. This results in the needle entering a lower tracheal space than desired (Figure 13.1) and may result in a lower placed tracheostomy tube (Figure 13.2). The longer tract may also make subsequent tube changes more difficult. The needle should be inserted at right angles to the approximate angle of the trachea towards the desired tracheal space. Only once in the tracheal lumen the needle should be angled

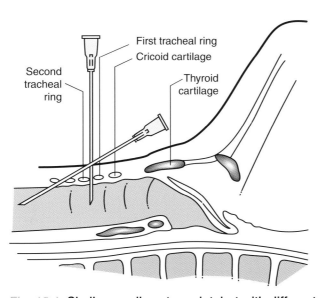

First tracheal ring
Cricoid cartilage
Second tracheal ring
Thyroid cartilage

Fig. 13.1 Similar needle entry point, but with different angulations, resulting in different spaces entered.

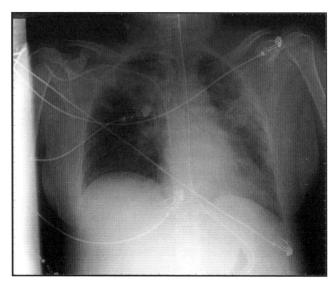

Fig. 13.2 **Low tracheostomy: the end of the tube is at the level of the carina.**

caudad. This is then followed by the advancement of the plastic cannula and subsequent insertion of the guidewire.

Green seeker needle

If difficulties are encountered in finding the tracheal lumen or achieving a midline needle placement then consider using a green needle as a seeker needle in a similar fashion to vascular access procedures. The sharp narrow diameter needle causes minimal bleeding and enters the trachea easily. Once correctly sited it is used as a guide for the larger introducing needle and cannula.

Transillumination with bronchoscope

A guide to the desired needle puncture site can be obtained by pressing anteriorly downwards with a finger or other blunt instrument and seeing the indentation of the anterior wall of the trachea via the bronchoscope. The illumination from the bronchoscope can also be seen on the anterior neck surface by angulating the scope towards the anterior tracheal wall at the desired tracheal space (Figure 13.3).

Avoid extreme neck extension

With the neck in extension, a larger portion of the trachea becomes extra-thoracic. This has implications for the siting of the skin incision

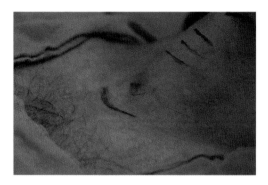

Fig. 13.3 **Transillumination with bronchoscope.**

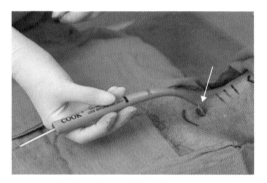

Fig. 13.4 **Tip of the Blue Rhino dilator is pulled right up against the 'collar' of the guiding catheter (arrow).**

and tracheal stoma, which will move in relation to each other in the neck. Hence the care should be taken to avoid extremes of extension during tracheostomy as on assuming a more neutral position the tracheal stoma may come to lie behind the sternum (Figure 13.2).

To ease insertion of dilators/tracheostomy

Pull end of dilator right up against the ridge on guiding catheter

Ensure the end of each dilator is pulled right up to the ridge (collar) on the 8 FG white guiding catheter to avoid any 'step' (Figure 13.4).

Aim for the space between tracheal rings

Aim for the space between tracheal rings and avoid hitting tracheal cartilages. If the site is too close to the tracheal cartilage, there is more chance of kinking the guidewire during dilatation. This may result on formation of a false passage and damage to tracheal

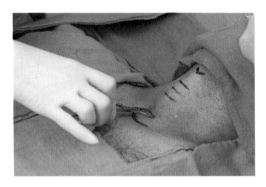

Fig. 13.5 **Blunt dissection with a pair of forceps.**

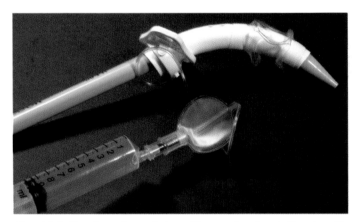

Fig. 13.6 **Tracheostomy tube with poorly streamlined cuff.**

cartilage rings, with the potential for tracheostomy cuff damage and increased risks of later tracheal stenosis.

Blunt dissection

A pair of Spencer Wells forceps or curved mosquito forceps is used for blunt dissection of the superficial muscle layers in a transverse plane (Figure 13.5). Vertical dilatation using the forceps will risk tearing the vessels. It is important *not* to dilate the trachea itself using the forceps because of the risk of tearing it. Any bleeding at this stage is much easier to control than when the trachea has been opened.

Streamline cuff

A poorly streamlined tracheostomy tube (Figure 13.6) is more difficult to insert through a tight stoma created by percutaneous

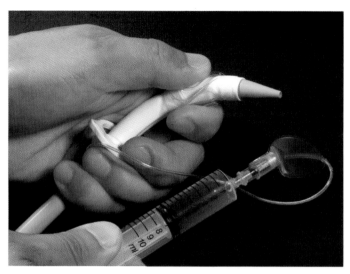

Fig. 13.7 **Trachoestomy tube with a streamlined cuff.**

dilatation. To ease insertion and to prevent cuff damage from sharp edges of cartilage, the cuff should be tapered back following the leak test for the cuff. First inflate the cuff and observe for any deflation from a leak over several minutes. Apply a generous layer of lubricating jelly (e.g. KY jelly). Then gently massage/milk the cuff away from the distal tip of the tracheostomy as the cuff is deflated (Figure 13.7). This procedure is easier if an assistant (non-sterile) can deflate the cuff.

Avoid 'step'
An appropriate tracheostomy tube must be selected for use with the loading dilator provided in the kit. An inappropriate tracheostomy tube when used with the loading dilator will result in a 'step', which will hinder the insertion (Figure 13.8). Using an appropriate tracheostomy tube on the dilator provided will minimise any 'step' or 'shoulder' (Figure 13.9).

Dilators and adjustable flange tubes
Current dilators are too short for most adjustable flange tracheostomy tubes. As a result there is minimal dilator protruding from the external end of the tube. This means that there it little to hold onto and problems ensue when attempts are made to adjust or remove the dilator (often with residual lubricant) from the tracheostomy tube following insertion. Clip an artery forceps onto the edge of the dilator and use it to adjust or remove the dilator.

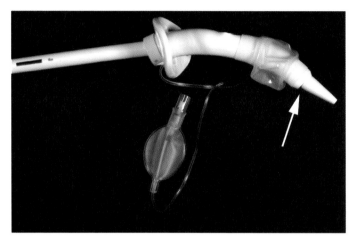

Fig. 13.8 An inappropriate tracheostomy tube (size 8) mounted on the 24 FG loading dilator of the Rüsch sequential dilator kit, resulting in a 'step' (arrow).

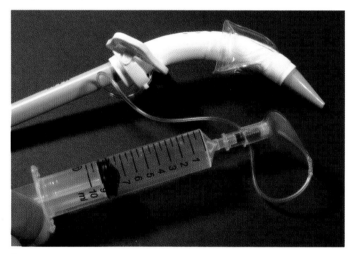

Fig. 13.9 An appropriate tracheostomy tube (size 8) mounted on the 28 FG loading dilator of the Blue Rhino kit, with no 'step'.

Preventing damage to the trachea

Aim for midline

Aim for midline cannulation to provide the maximal antero-posterior diameter to reduce the chance of posterior tracheal wall trauma.
A midline stoma, at right angles to the trachea, at a reasonable level in the neck, provides the shortest direct route to the trachea, which should make subsequent tube changes easier and less traumatic.

Continuous visualisation of the procedure with a bronchoscope

Continuous visualisation throughout the procedure, including during the dilatation process, should minimise damage to the tracheal ring cartilages and posterior tracheal wall.

Monitor the tracheostomy tube cuff pressure

Keeping the cuff pressure below 25 cm H_2O (18 mmHg) will minimise tracheal mucosa ischaemia and reduce the risk of tracheal stenosis in the future. When inflating the cuff the minimum volume should be used to prevent air leaks. A 10 ml syringe is used to gradually inflate the cuff at 0.5 ml increments. A stethoscope is placed just below the thyroid cartilage to listen for any air leaks. Do not rely on normal hearing. A stethoscope is required for accuracy. Estimation of cuff pressure by fingertip pressure on the external pilot balloon is inaccurate. There are commercially available devices to monitor such pressures (see page 65).

Weaning failure

In patients with large amounts of viscous secretions, a possible explanation for failure to wean may be due to the increased work of breathing due to a narrowed tracheostomy lumen by biofilm, and dried mucus build up (Figure 13.10). It is mucus rather than this biofilm, which causes significant narrowing.

e.g. size 8 tracheostomy tube (ID 8 mm)

Flow $\propto$ radius^4
Therefore 1 mm biofilm will reduce the radius from 4 mm to 3 mm
Flow $= 4^4 = 256$
Flow $= 3^4 = 81$
Reduction in flow $= (256 - 81)/256 = 175/256 = 68\%$

Prevention of tracheostomy tube blockage

Possible solutions include adequate humidification, nebulised acetylcysteine, changing the tube more frequently or selecting a tube with an inner cannula.

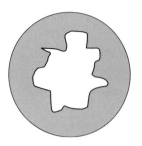

Fig. 13.10 Tracheostomy tube lumen in section with a thick mucus/biofilm lining.

Repeat percutaneous tracheostomy

The role of percutaneous techniques for revision procedures in tracheostomy has never been formally evaluated. This includes both previous open and percutaneous procedures. Common sense would dictate that the amount of further dissection of tissue should be minimised and potentially ischaemic bridges of skin or trachea should be avoided for fear of further tissue breakdown. On this basis it seems sensible to open up the old scar by either blunt dissection or serial dilation. It is sensible to perform endoscopy first to make sure any instruments pass through the old scar rather than immediately above or below it, and to look for any pre-existing stenosis or other problems. In the presence of significant pre-existing damage, consider referral for open procedure. In the first few weeks following tracheostomy, stomas require little force to be opened with artery forceps or percutaneous dilators.

It should be noted that vessels and other structures which are not traditionally near the trachea may become adherent to the trachea following surgery, e.g. open tracheostomy with extensive scarring or thyroidectomy procedures.

Difficulties in finding an existing tract down into the trachea

This is a common problem, particularly in the patient with a thicker neck or when there have been repeated attempts at recannulation, which open up false tissue tracts. The following manoeuvres may help:

- Do not be frightened to put your finger into the stoma and feel your way down into the tissues. You can usually feel the hole in the rigid trachea to give a guide as to its position.

- Alternatively, use a bronchoscope to view from the inside to visualise the stoma and use a blunt instrument e.g. artery forceps, to probe around, looking for distortion of the anterior tracheal wall to give a clue as to where the forceps are, and move appropriately until the forceps appear in the trachea. The guidewire and stiffening plastic sheath can then be passed alongside the forceps into the trachea and the tract dilated up in the usual fashion.

The patient with the short fat neck

Regrettably, many patients requiring ventilatory support on intensive care unit (ICU) will be obese, elderly, with vertebral collapse and a hyper-inflated chest. The net effect of all these findings is an overall shortening of the neck. Palpation reveals a very short distance between the sternal notch and the cricoid cartilage. Palpate and feel the backwards angle of the trachea, particularly in the older patient.

It is therefore impossible to get into the lower tracheal cartilages without the tracheal puncture site being retrosternal. A retrosternal puncture site should be avoided to avoid difficulties in recannulation even if the original tube could be inserted without difficulty. In such cases a balanced decision needs to be made about the site of access to the trachea, and it may be necessary to go between the cricoid or the first ring, or even through the cricothyroid membrane if all else fails. Note that the great vessels, across the midline, will be in the usual place just behind the sternum.

An example is illustrated in Figures 13.11–13.13. This patient underwent a successful elective abdominal aortic aneurysm repair but suffered a severe postoperative cerebrovascular accident. He had two failed extubations, due to severe stridor caused by glottic oedema and vocal cord palsy. Open surgical tracheostomy was deemed to be difficult without resection of the sternum and also the thyroid gland covered the short segment of the trachea that was exposed in the neck (Figure 13.12). Sternal resection is a major procedure, which could increase the risk of erosion of the tube into the innominate vessels. The resection would also involve taking out the sterno-clavicular joints, which could interfere with the respiratory

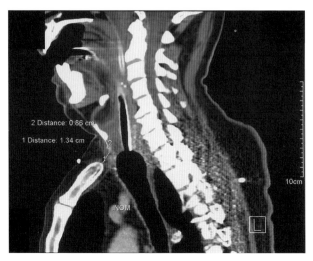

Fig. 13.11 Sagittal computed tomography (CT) image showing the very narrow cricoid to sternal distance (1.34 cm) and the cricothyroid space (0.86 cm). Note the proximity of the innominate vessels to the trachea behind the sternum (INOM). This followed collapsed thoracic vertebrae and hyperinflated lungs from chronic obstructive pulmonary disease (COPD).

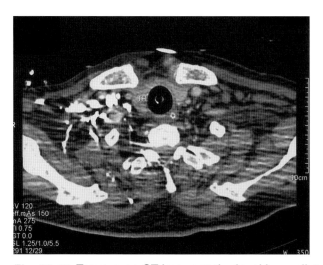

Fig. 13.12 Transverse CT image at the level immediately above the sternum (just shown as line of bone between two medial ends of clavicles), showing the thyroid gland enveloping the trachea (TH).

dynamics and affect weaning. A cricothyroidotomy with a Melker cuffed tube was seen as the safest option to avoid trauma to the thyroid but still able to provide positive ventilation and a protected airway, to facilitate weaning. This was performed successfully by one

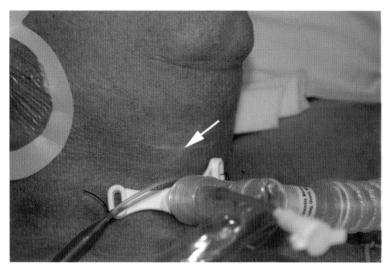

Fig. 13.13 The same patient as Figures 13.11 and 13.12, post-cricothyroidotomy. There are two anterior neck scars, one from previous neck abscess drainage (arrow) and one from a parathyroidectomy (hidden by the flange of the tube).

of the authors (Henry G.W. Paw) after 24 days of translaryngeal intubation (Figure 13.13).

Ways to reduce bleeding

Identify vessels and the thyroid gland using ultrasound before each procedure

To provide a better picture of the veins, the patient may have to be tipped head down or perform a Valsalva procedure if able. Remember not to press too firmly with the ultrasound probe as this will compress the vein.

Head up tilt of up to 30°

This will prevent venous engorgement and minimise the risk of vessel damage.

Minimise size of skin incisions

Skin incisions should be as small (usually 1.5 cm) as required to allow the passage of the dilator. A stoma, which provides the tracheostomy tube with a snug fit, will provide tamponade to bleeding vessels.

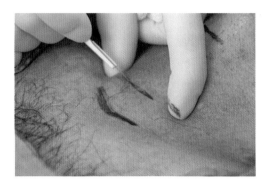

Fig. 13.14 **Skin incision.**

Minimise depth of skin incisions

The skin incision should be just skin deep (Figure 13.14). Any deeper and you may cut into vessels, e.g. anterior jugular veins.

Digital pressure or dilator tamponade

Press on skin tissues above and below to control venous bleeding. Pack the wound with gauze ribbon or an unfolded gauze swab and compress, and re-examine the wound later when bleeding has usually stopped.

Tie-off bleeding points

It may be difficult to identify a bleeding point in the small stoma. Consider using a transfixion stitch through the tissues in the area of bleeding.

Check airway for blood clots if the trachea has been opened and leave the bronchoscope at the bedside to recheck later in the day.

Indications for surgical referral

These include:

- A failed procedure due to bleeding and an ongoing need for tracheostomy.
- Persistent bleeding, in particular if there is suspected great vein/artery damage: there is significant risk of secondary bleeding, hours/days later.

- Difficulties in passing tubes or dilators, a tissue flap may be present.
- Persistent air leaks.
- Significant tracheal wall damage.

Achieving a better cosmetic scar

Small skin incision

The skin incision should be as small as required to allow the passage of the dilator. A snugger fit of skin around the tracheostomy tube reduces the exposure in the tracheostomy wound. This might explain the lower rates of stomal infection with percutaneous tracheostomy, which will produce a better cosmetic result after healing.

Horizonatal skin incision

The authors are aware that some operators prefer a vertical incision in the mistaken belief that the midline is avascular. As shown in previous chapters, the midline is not always avascular. Horizontal incision along the Langerhan's line will improve wound healing and achieve a better cosmetic result.

Audit Form for Recording Percutaneous Tracheostomy

Percutaneous Tracheostomy
York Hospital

Patient addressograph: Number:
                                                          Date:

Operator:

Fibreoptic bronchoscopist:

Relevant medical history:

Reason for tracheostomy:
    Anticipated slow wean
    Slow wean
    Failed extubation
    Others

Days intubated prior to tracheostomy:

ABG prior to tracheostomy
    FiO_2:
    PaO_2:
    $PaCO_2$:

Ventilation mode:
PS:
CPAP/PEEP:

Clotting screen: INR   APPT   Platelets

Technique: Cooks (Ciaglia)   Rüsch (PercuQuick)   Rhino

Tracheostomy tube: TRACOE   Tracheostomy tube size:
                      Portex (blue line)
                      TracheoSoft (Perc)
                      Shiley (non-fenestrated)
                      Rüsch

Is Ultrasound Scan used before procedure?
Difficulties during procedure/complications:
Date tracheostomy decannulated:

Audit Form for Recording Surgical Open Tracheostomy

Surgical Tracheostomy
York Hospital

Number: Date:

Patient addressograph:

Operator:

ASA:

Relevant medical history:

Reason(s) for referral to surgeons:

Days intubated prior to tracheostomy:

ABG prior to tracheostomy
    FiO_2:
    PaO_2:
    $PaCO_2$:

Ventilation mode:
PS:
CPAP/PEEP:

Clotting screen: INR   APPT   Platelets

Duration (from skin incision to trachy placement):   min

Tracheostomy tube size:

CXR findings:

Complications:

Date tracheostomy decannulated:

Blue Dye Test

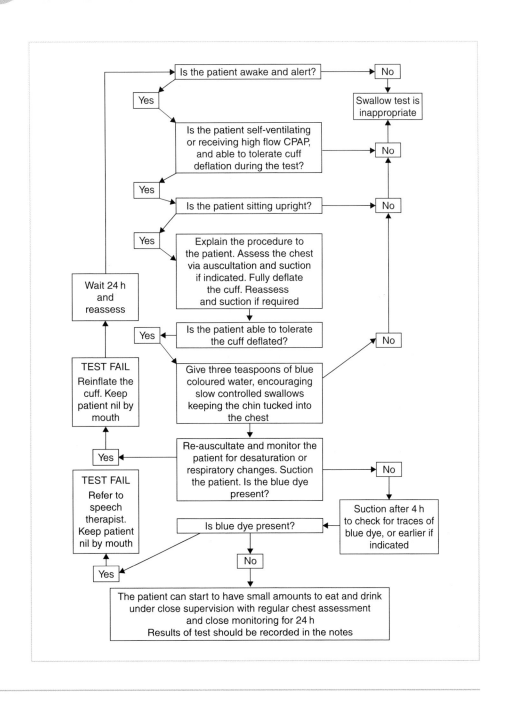

Index

Page numbers in *italics* refer to figures; note that figures are only indicated when they are separated from their text references.